The Ethics of Embryonic Stem Cell Research

ISSUES IN BIOMEDICAL ETHICS

General Editors
John Harris and Søren Holm

Consulting Editors
Raanan Gillon and Bonnie Steinbock

The late twentieth century witnessed dramatic technological developments in biomedical science and in the delivery of healthcare, and these developments have brought with them important social changes. All too often ethical analysis has lagged behind these changes. The purpose of this series is to provide lively, up-to-date, and authoritative studies for the increasingly large and diverse readership concerned with issues in biomedical ethics—not just healthcare trainees and professionals, but also philosophers, social scientists, lawyers, social workers, and legislators. The series will feature both single-author and multi-author books, short and accessible enough to be widely read, each of them focused on an issue of outstanding current importance and interest. Philosophers, doctors, and lawyers from a number of countries feature among the authors lined up for the series.

The Ethics of
Embryonic Stem
Cell Research

Katrien Devolder

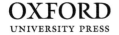
OXFORD
UNIVERSITY PRESS

OXFORD
UNIVERSITY PRESS

Great Clarendon Street, Oxford, OX2 6DP,
United Kingdom

Oxford University Press is a department of the University of Oxford.
It furthers the University's objective of excellence in research, scholarship,
and education by publishing worldwide. Oxford is a registered trade mark of
Oxford University Press in the UK and in certain other countries

First Edition published in 2015

Impression: 1

Published in the United States of America by Oxford University Press
198 Madison Avenue, New York, NY 10016, United States of America

British Library Cataloguing in Publication Data
Data available

Library of Congress Control Number: 2014942175

ISBN 978-0-19-954799-9

Printed and bound by
CPI Group (UK) Ltd, Croydon, CR0 4YY

Acknowledgements

Writing a book is a demanding undertaking, and I could not have brought this project to a good end without the support of a number of people.

I am very grateful for the opportunities John Harris has given me throughout the years, including the opportunity to contribute to this book series. I thank him for his confidence in me, as well as for his patience, as it took somewhat longer than I expected to finish this book.

I would also like to thank those who read drafts of this work: Tom Douglas gave me several rounds of helpful comments on drafts of the whole manuscript, and these have greatly improved this book; Sam Kerstein, Jeff McMahan, Chris Megone, Freddy Mortier, Russell Powell, and Jonny Pugh offered very valuable comments on precursors to Chapter 2; Tim Davies read parts of the manuscript to check the accuracy of the scientific claims I make. (If any mistakes in the science remain they are, of course, of my own doing.) I would also like to thank Willy Lensch whose explanations of various aspects of stem cell science have been of great benefit to me. The anonymous reviewers of this book gave me much constructive feedback that helped me improve the manuscript, for which I am grateful. Parts of the book have been presented as papers at conferences and seminars, and I have profited a great deal from the comments and questions received from the audience.

The research required to write this book was generously funded by Ghent University and the Research Foundation Flanders (FWO). The Brocher Foundation in Switzerland also supported this project by awarding me a 'residency' scholarship. I have very fond memories of my stay there and would like to thank the staff for providing such a wonderful environment for academics who wish to immerse themselves in a particular project. I am also greatly indebted to Julian Savulescu and Dan Brock, who gave me the opportunity to spend time at, respectively, the Oxford Uehiro Centre for Practical Ethics and the Harvard University Program in Ethics & Health. Working in such stimulating and challenging intellectual environments contributed substantially to the quality of this work. I also wish to thank Antoine and Sylvie Winckler for their generosity. I would write another book simply to be able to work in such a wonderful setting again!

I drew on a number of published papers in writing this book, although in most cases the material was substantially reworked. These papers are: 'Killing Discarded Embryos and the Nothing-is-Lost Principle', *Journal of Applied Philosophy*, 30/4 (2013); 'Embryo Deaths in Reproduction and Embryo Research: A Reply to Murphy's Double Effect Argument', *Journal of Medical Ethics*, 39/8 (2013); 'Against the Discarded-Created Distinction in Embryonic Stem Cell Research', in M. Quigley, S. Chan, and J. Harris (eds), *Stem Cells: New Frontiers in Science and Ethics* (World Scientific Publishing, 2012); 'Complicity in Stem Cell Research: The Case of Induced Pluripotent Stem Cells', *Human Reproduction*, 25/9 (2010); 'To Be or Not to Be? Are Induced Pluripotent Stem Cells Potential Babies, and does it Matter?', *EMBO Reports*, 10/12 (2009); 'Rescuing Human Embryonic Stem Cell Research: The Possibility of Embryo Reconstitution', *Metaphilosophy*, 28/2–3 (2007); 'What's in a Name? Embryos, Entities and ANTities in the Stem Cell Debate', *Journal of Medical Ethics* 2006, 32/1 (2006); and 'Creating and Sacrificing Embryos for Stem Cells', *Journal of Medical Ethics*, 31/6 (2005).

Writing a book requires hard work and I could never have finished it without many fun moments in between. Many thanks to all my friends, and especially to Lot, Ellen, Liza, and Zus for all the good laughs. Thanks so much to my parents, who are my biggest supporters and are always there to help me in any way they can. And finally, thanks to Tom who has not only diverted me in stressful moments, but has also always strongly supported and encouraged me throughout the whole writing process. His confidence in me gave me the courage to complete this book.

Katrien Devolder

Ghent
18 February 2014

Contents

1

Introduction
The Ethics of Embryonic Stem Cell Research

1.1. The Problem

The main controversy surrounding stem cell research is not about *whether* we should use stem cells for research and therapeutic purposes—virtually everyone agrees we should—but about *what source* of stem cells we should use, and how we should obtain them. It is only the isolation and use of stem cells from early human embryos that has set off a storm of controversy and has resulted in one of the most contentious debates in bioethics: the human embryonic stem cell debate.

Most of the ethical debate about human embryonic stem cell research turns on a fundamental disagreement about how we should treat early human embryos. As it is currently done, the isolation of human embryonic stem cells involves a process in which an early embryo is destroyed. Many people accord a significant moral status to the human embryo and think that it may never simply be used in whatever way suits our research interests. Some think that human embryos (henceforth just 'embryos'—I will indicate when I refer to non-human embryos) should never be harmed or destroyed in scientific research that is not to their own benefit. At the same time there is wide agreement that embryonic stem cell research holds unique promise for developing therapies for currently incurable diseases and conditions, and for important biomedical research. It is believed that embryonic stem cell research could prevent a great amount of suffering and could improve and prolong many people's lives. This has resulted in what I will, throughout the book, refer to as

The Problem. Either one supports embryonic stem cell research and accepts resulting embryo destruction, or one opposes embryonic stem cell research and accepts that the potential benefits of this research will be foregone.

The Problem consists of a choice between two options, where, whatever option one takes, and however clear it is that one should take that particular option, one's choice will involve a significant cost as the conflicting but important value is left unsatisfied.

Of course, not everyone is confronted with the Problem. For those who believe an early embryo is merely a collection of cells, the fact that embryonic stem cell research involves destroying embryos provides no moral reason to abstain from such research. However, for those who believe the embryo has a significant moral status the Problem is very real.[1]

In this book I do not offer an exhaustive overview of all the ethical issues raised by embryonic stem cell research. I focus squarely on the Problem as it has been at the centre of the embryonic stem cell debate. Responses to the Problem have greatly influenced the regulation of stem cell research, and thus, the course this research has taken. There have been two major types of response. The first type of response has been to adopt a middle-ground position—a position between the dominant opposing views on the permissibility of embryonic stem cell research. The two dominant opposing views hold respectively that all embryonic stem cell research is morally unacceptable and that embryonic stem cell research is no more problematic than other kinds of research in cell biology. By contrast, middle-ground positions—positions between these two views—distinguish between different types or aspects of embryonic stem cell research, accepting some but not others. The second type of response to the Problem has been the development of technical solutions. Several techniques have been proposed to enable researchers to obtain embryonic stem cells, or their functional equivalents, without harming or destroying embryos.

Before I proceed with further introducing these two types of response, I should first explain the Problem in more detail. Two questions arise: (1) what moral reasons, if any, are there to support embryonic stem cell research?, and (2) what moral reasons, if any, are there to oppose it?

---

[1] Those who think we have moral reason to defend an ethical position that incorporates others' reasonable views may also be faced with the Problem. I will come back to this issue in Chapter 5.

1.2. Reasons for Supporting Embryonic Stem Cell Research

Beneficence

Support for embryonic stem cell research has sometimes been grounded in considerations of freedom of research[2] and scientific progress.[3] However, the main reason for supporting embryonic stem cell research is that it is expected to help us prevent and treat devastating diseases and disability. Failing to pursue embryonic stem cell research can be expected to result in much avoidable suffering and many premature deaths. It is widely accepted that we have significant moral reasons to benefit people if we can and to prevent avoidable suffering and premature death. These are reasons of beneficence.[4] The view that there are such reasons of beneficence does not rely on controversial theoretical assumptions. Indeed, it could be accepted by the proponents of all of the leading ethical theories. Plausibly, then, there are significant moral reasons for pursuing embryonic stem cell research. However, to substantiate the claim that there are such reasons, more needs to be said about what stem cells are and why they are believed to be so important.

Stem cells

Stem cells are undifferentiated cells, which means that they have not yet been committed to become 'specialized cells', that is, cells with a specific function, such as heart cells, liver cells or skin cells. The combination of two properties make stem cells different from any other type of cell in our body: (1) the capacity for continued replication while maintaining their undifferentiated state (this sort of replication is called 'proliferation' or 'self-renewal') and (2) the capacity to differentiate into various cell

---

[2] See e.g. ESHRE Taskforce on Ethics and Law, 'Stem Cells', *Human Reproduction*, 17 (2002), 1409–10. Thomas Heinemann and Ludger Honnefelder, 'Principles of Ethical Decision Making Regarding Embryonic Stem Cell Research in Germany', *Bioethics*, 16 (2002), 530–43. Davor Solter et al., *Embryo Research in Pluralistic Europe* (Berlin and Heidelberg: Springer-Verlag, 2003), 142.

[3] See e.g. Deutsche Forschungsgemeinschaft (German Research Foundation), 'New DFG Recommendations Concerning Research with Human Stem Cells', press release 16 (3 May 2001).

[4] Tom L. Beauchamp and James F. Childress, *Principles of Biomedical Ethics* (New York: Oxford University Press, 2001).

types of the body. One mechanism by which stem cells can replicate is asymmetric cell division, whereby a stem cell divides, producing one daughter cell like itself—a stem cell—and another more specialized daughter cell, ready for further specialization. But stem cells can also divide symmetrically. Both daughter cells will then acquire the same cell fate, and will be either stem cells or differentiated—that is, somewhat specialized—cells.

The importance of stem cells cannot be underestimated. All our body cells stem from stem cells (hence the name). In fact, each of us was once a stem cell (at least, if it is true that each of us was once a zygote[5]). A zygote is a stem cell par excellence. It is totipotent, which means that it can give rise to all the cells of the developing organism, including the placenta and other supporting tissues. After a few cycles of cell division, some cells are committed to forming the 'embryo proper', as opposed to the supporting tissues. These cells are thus somewhat more specialized than the zygote and the cells of the very early embryo. Because they can give rise to any of our body cells (and thus to all our fluids, tissues, and organs), but not the placenta and other supporting tissues, they are referred to as pluripotent stem cells. As the embryo develops further these cells will become increasingly specialized and will thus lose their pluripotency. They will become multipotent and will only be able to give rise to some types of body cell (for example, only to all types of blood cell).

Stem cells play a crucial role in our earliest development, but they are also essential later in life. Some of our organs and tissues still contain stem cells. They regularly divide and differentiate to replenish dying cells in tissues that must perpetually renew, such as the blood or the gut, and to regenerate tissues and organs that are damaged. Stem cells provide a constant supply of replacement cells, thereby serving as a repair system for the body. However, not all tissues and organs contain stem cells and not all stem cells present in the body start dividing and differentiating when an organ or tissue are damaged. The liver, for

---

[5] A zygote is the cell formed when a sperm fertilizes an egg. Each of us developed from a zygote, but some deny that we ever *were* zygotes (just like we were never oocytes), holding that we did not come to exist until some later point in embryonic development. See e.g. Jeff McMahan, *The Ethics of Killing: Problems at the Margins of Life* (New York: Oxford University Press, 2002).

example, regenerates quite well in response to damage, but the heart does not. This is unfortunate. If all our organs and tissues could regenerate, we could continuously repair our body and live much longer and healthier lives. This is where stem cell research comes into play: it may help us achieve this goal.

Stem cell-based therapies

One major goal of stem cell research is the development of stem cell-based therapies. The capacity of stem cells to proliferate and differentiate into various cell types of the body makes them extremely useful tools for therapy.

One stem cell-based therapy that has been routine for decades is bone marrow transplantation for the treatment of leukaemia and other blood disorders. In the 1950s, scientists discovered that bone marrow contains haematopoietic stem cells, which can give rise to all types of blood cell. Bone marrow transplantation involves the intravenous injection of these haematopoietic stem cells into a patient whose blood cells are severely reduced, or have been destroyed by high doses of chemotherapy or irradiation. The transplanted stem cells 'home' into the patient's bone marrow where they start to generate blood cells, thus replenishing the patient's blood and immune system.

Scientists interested in the therapeutic benefits of stem cells focus on two main approaches. An initial approach is to produce stem cell-derived replacement cells in the laboratory. The idea is that if a damaged tissue or organ cannot repair itself, stem cells could be obtained elsewhere. There are different sources of stem cells. Since the discovery and isolation of haematopoietic stem cells from the bone marrow, stem cells have been derived from many other organs and tissues, including peripheral blood and umbilical cord blood, placental tissues, the brain, gum tissue, the epithelia (outer layers) of the skin and digestive system, the cornea, retina, liver, teeth, and testes. Stem cells from organs and tissues from individuals after birth are *adult* stem cells, sometimes also referred to as somatic stem cells. Stem cells have also been isolated from the gametes (egg or sperm cells), tissues, and organs from aborted foetuses. These are usually referred to as *foetal* stem cells. (Note that foetal stem cells are sometimes categorized as adult stem cells, since they share many of the same features.) Finally, stem cells have been isolated from the inner cell mass of early embryos. In 1998, James Thomson's research group at the University of Wisconsin was the first to isolate and culture such *embryonic* stem cells.[6]

If a damaged tissue or organ cannot repair itself, stem cells could be obtained from these different stem cell sources. Scientists could then culture these stem cells by creating conditions that enable them to replicate many times in a petri dish without differentiating. Such a population of proliferating stem cells originating from a single parent group of stem cells is a stem cell line. Stem cells from this stem cell line could then be coaxed to differentiate into the desired cell type, and be transferred into the patient so that they can repair the damaged tissue or organ. For example, stem cells obtained from early embryos could be induced to differentiate into cardiomyocytes (heart muscle cells) to repair or replace damaged heart tissue, into insulin-producing cells to treat diabetes, or into neurons and their supporting tissues to repair spinal cord injuries. In 2010, Geron (a California based biotechnology company) conducted the first phase-I clinical trial with embryonic stem cells. Embryonic stem cell-derived oligodendrocyte progenitor cells were injected directly into the lesion site of patients with acute spinal cord injury. Oligodendrocytes are cells which support nerve cells. They can be lost in spinal cord injury, resulting in loss of myelin and neuronal function, which causes paralysis. Other clinical trials with embryonic stem cells are aimed at the development of an embryonic stem cell therapy for a rare form of juvenile blindness. The aim is to provide the patient with retinal pigment epithelium cells derived from embryonic stem cells to restore their vision.[7]

If scientists fully understood, and were able to replicate, the body's mechanisms for inducing cell differentiation, they could create whole tissues or even organs in the laboratory. There have already been reports of successful transplantation of skin, bladders, and sections of windpipes generated partly by stem cell-derived replacement cells. For example, in 2008, a woman received a new bronchus (a section of the respiratory

[6] James A. Thomson et al., 'Embryonic Stem Cell Lines Derived from Human Blastocysts', *Science*, 282 (1998), 1145–7.

[7] Raymond D. Lund, et al., 'Human Embryonic Stem Cell-Derived Cells Rescue Visual Function in Dystrophic RCS Rats', *Cloning and Stem Cells*, 8 (2006), 189–99. Bin Lu et al., 'Long-Term Safety and Function of RPE from Human Embryonic Stem Cells in Preclinical Models of Macular Degeneration', *Stem Cells*, 27 (2009), 2126–35.

tract) generated in part from her own stem cells.[8] A bronchus from a deceased donor was first stripped of cells that could cause immune reaction in the recipient and was subsequently populated with cartilage and epithelial cells produced in the laboratory from the woman's own haematopoietic stem cells. The bronchus was then successfully transplanted into the woman. Research is also being conducted into combining this sort of stem cell-based therapy with gene therapy. For example, scientists hope to treat cystic fibrosis by first inducing the patient's haematopoietic stem cells (cells that normally produce blood cells) to differentiate into airway-lining epithelial cells and then to correct, in these cells, the genetic defect that causes airway blockage in patients with cystic fibrosis. These genetically modified cells could then restore a cellular function essential to keeping the airways clear of mucus and airborne irritants.[9]

The second approach to developing stem cell-based treatments involves triggering stem cells already present in the body to migrate to and repair damaged tissues and organs.[10] Transplanted stem cells or artificial scaffolds that release biochemical factors could spur stem cells already present in the body into action. These techniques have been used in clinical trials to stimulate bone growth, cartilage, growth and heart repair. For example, a research team from Northwestern University in Chicago designed a biological material that activates bone marrow stem cells in the body to produce natural cartilage that can repair joints.[11]

Stem cell research may open up radically new ways of treating currently untreatable diseases, disorders, and injuries. Unlike currently available drugs, which mainly treat or delay symptoms, stem cells could enable us to repair or even replace damaged tissues or organs. Thus, stem cells are an extremely promising tool for regenerative medicine. However, at the time of writing, most stem cell-based therapies are

---

[8] Paolo Macchiarini et al., 'Clinical Transplantation of a Tissue-Engineered Airway', *The Lancet*, 372 (2008), 2023–30.

[9] Maurilio Sampaolesi et al., 'Mesoangioblast Stem Cells Ameliorate Muscle Function in Dystrophic Dogs', *Nature*, 444 (2006), 574–9.

[10] Gitte S. Jensen and Christian Drapeau, 'The Use of in situ Bone Marrow Stem Cells for the Treatment of Various Degenerative Diseases', *Medical Hypotheses*, 59 (2002), 422–8.

[11] Ramille N. Shah et al., 'Supramolecular Design of Self-Assembling Nanofibers for Cartilage Regeneration', *Proceedings of the National Academy of Sciences*, 107 (2010), 3293–8.

still in the experimental stage. Before therapeutic applications can be realized, many technical hurdles need to be overcome and many questions need to be answered, including basic questions about the mechanisms of proliferation, cell migration, and differentiation.

Biomedical research

In addition to their therapeutic promise, stem cells are potentially powerful tools for biomedical research. Scientists may be able to learn about mechanisms regulating cell growth, migration, and differentiation by observing stem cells that have been induced to differentiate into different types of body cell. A better understanding of these mechanisms could provide insight into early human development and into how tissues are maintained throughout life. It could also help us to explain how and why things sometimes go wrong in the development process, for example, in birth defects. Other major uses of stem cells in biomedical research include the creation of *in vitro* models for the study of diseases and for drug discovery and toxicity testing. Diseases could be studied or drugs could be tested on stem cells and their derivatives in a petri dish, rather than in live persons or animals. This could considerably increase the efficiency of these studies and tests, and make them safer. For example, testing the toxicity of candidate drug therapies on stem cells and their derivatives in a petri dish would avoid dangerous exposure of patients to sometimes highly experimental drugs (see section 2.1).

There is wide agreement in the scientific community that stem cell research holds the potential to significantly benefit a large number of people. It could not only prolong people's lives, but also considerably reduce morbidity. Failing to pursue this research is expected to result in many premature deaths and much avoidable suffering. As mentioned earlier, it is widely accepted that we have significant moral reason to benefit people if we can and to prevent avoidable suffering and premature death. There are thus significant reasons of beneficence for pursuing stem cell research.

However, embryonic stem cell research is but one strand of stem cell research. Are there also moral reasons for pursuing this controversial type of stem cell research in particular?

Why embryonic stem cells?

Not all types of stem cells are the same, and the differences between embryonic, foetal, and adult stem cells confer advantages and disadvantages for different uses. There is as yet no consensus on the exact characteristics and the potential of the different types of stem cell, but there is wide agreement on the following.

First, in a technical sense, embryonic stem cells are typically easier to obtain than foetal and adult stem cells. (Since foetal stem cells share many properties with adult stem cells, I will no longer mention them separately.) Embryonic stem cells are derived from embryos at the blastocyst stage. At that stage the embryo is mainly a hollow ball the size of a pinhead, with a small inner cell mass (there are no organs or blood yet—only a cluster of inner cell mass cells). A blastocyst consists of 125–250 cells, of which the inner cell mass comprises between 27 and 45 cells. Using microsurgery, researchers first remove the embryo's inner cell mass cells and then culture these cells in the laboratory to form an embryonic stem cell line. The microsurgical procedure is so invasive that it destroys the embryo's structure, thereby impeding the embryo's further development. What remains of the embryo is discarded. The procedure for deriving embryonic stem cells is relatively efficient, though derivation efficiency varies between different laboratories. Adult stem cells are generally more difficult to isolate because they are only present in small numbers. In mouse bone marrow, for example, one in 10,000 cells is a stem cell, and in humans the ratio may be even lower. Adult stem cells are also often hard, if not impossible, to harvest from the patient's organs and tissues, for example, from difficult to access organs like the heart or the brain. In most tissues there is no particular location in which stem cells can reliably be found and techniques to identify them are not efficient. Moreover, many tissues may not contain stem cells at all.

A second significant advantage of embryonic over adult stem cells is that they have a much greater proliferation capacity. Embryonic stem cells multiply readily. Under the right culture conditions they can proliferate indefinitely. With most adult stem cells, on the other hand, proliferation is slow and difficult to induce. A restricted proliferation capacity typically has negative implications for research and therapeutic applications as both require sufficient numbers of stem cells.

A third, and perhaps the most important, advantage of embryonic stem cells over adult stem cells is that they are more versatile. Embryonic stem cells are *pluripotent*: they can (in theory) give rise to all cell types of the body. Numerous studies have demonstrated the differentiation potential of embryonic stem cells *in vitro*. For example, embryonic stem cells have been induced to give rise to neural progenitors, insulin-producing cells, cardiomyocytes, and endothelial cells.[12] Their enormous plasticity makes embryonic stem cells useful tools for a wide array of therapeutic applications. In the mouse there is proof of concept for the use of embryonic stem cells to treat various models of diseases and conditions, including diabetes, Parkinson's disease, myocardial infarction, and spinal cord injury.[13] The plasticity of embryonic stem cells also has major advantages for biomedical research including for drug discovery and toxicity testing.

Adult stem cells are believed to be much less versatile than embryonic stem cells. They are *multipotent*, which means they can differentiate to yield only a limited number of cell types, typically the cell types from the area in the body where they were located. For example, skin stem cells can give rise to epidermal cells (cells making up the outer layer of the skin), keratinocytes (cells responsible for producing the keratin layer in our skin, which protects it from environmental damage such as UV), and hair follicles; and haematopoietic stem cells found in the blood can give rise to all the types of blood cell. Some studies suggest that adult stem cells may have greater plasticity than originally thought. For example,

---

[12] Benjamin E. Reubinoff et al., 'Embryonic Stem Cell Lines from Human Blastocysts: Somatic Differentiation in Vitro', *Nature Biotechnology*, 18 (2000), 399–404. Suheir Assady et al., 'Insulin Production by Human Embryonic Stem Cells', *Diabetes*, 50 (2001), 1691–7. Izhak Kehat et al., 'Human Embryonic Stem Cells Can Differentiate into Myocytes with Structural and Functional Properties of Cardiomyocytes', *Journal of Clinical Investigation*, 108 (2001), 407–14. Shulamit Levenberg et al., 'Endothelial Cells Derived from Human Embryonic Stem Cells', *Proceedings of the National Academy of Sciences USA*, 99 (2002), 4391–6.

[13] John W. McDonald et al., 'Transplanted Embryonic Stem Cells Survive, Differentiate and Promote Recovery in Injured Rat Spinal Cord', *Nature Medicine*, 5 (1999), 1410–12. Bernat Soria et al., 'Insulin-Secreting Cells Derived from Embryonic Stem Cells Normalize Glycemia in Streptozotocin-Induced Diabetic Mice', *Diabetes*, 49 (2000), 157–62. Jong-Hoon Kim et al., 'Dopamine Neurons Derived from Embryonic Stem Cells Function in an Animal Model of Parkinson's Disease', *Nature*, 418 (2002), 50–6. Jiang-Yong Min et al., 'Transplantation of Embryonic Stem Cells Improves Cardiac Function in Postinfarcted Rats', *Journal of Applied Physiology*, 92 (2002), 288–96.

one study showed that stem cells from the amniotic fluid could give rise to many types of functioning body cells.[14] However, these stem cells were still less versatile than embryonic stem cells. A restricted capacity to differentiate limits the potential applications of adult stem cells.

Embryonic stem cells also have some disadvantages compared to adult stem cells. Their capacities for proliferation and differentiation increase the risk that, after transplantation, the stem cells will cause tumour formation in the patient's body. There is no strong evidence for such a risk with adult stem cells. However, several strategies have been proposed to reduce that risk, including differentiating embryonic stem cells in long-term cultures before transfer.[15]

Another important disadvantage of embryonic stem cells over adult stem cells is that they will normally not be genetically identical to the patient. Whereas adult stem cells can be harvested from the patient (though, given the restrictions mentioned, this may not always be possible), embryonic stem cells would normally be allogeneic (genetically different) cells as they are typically derived from embryos donated for research after *in vitro* fertilization (IVF) treatment (see section 2.1). Because these stem cells would have a genetic identity different from that of the recipient—the patient—they may, when used in therapy, be rejected by her immune system. Immunorejection can occur when the recipient's body does not recognize the transplanted cells, tissues, or organs as its own and as a defence mechanism attempts to destroy them. Another type of immunorejection involves a condition called graft-versus-host disease, in which immune cells contaminating the graft recognize the new host—the patient—as foreign and attack the host's tissues and organs. Both types of immunorejection can result in loss of the transplanted material and potentially the death of the patient. It is one of the most serious problems faced in transplant surgery.

To overcome problems of immunorejection of embryonic stem cells and their derivatives, a number of solutions have been proposed,[16] including

---

[14] Dafni Moschidou et al., 'Valproic Acid Confers Functional Pluripotency to Human Amniotic Fluid Stem Cells in a Transgene-Free Approach', *Molecular Therapy*, 20 (2012), 1953–67.

[15] Rita Pilar Cervera and Miodrag Stojkovic, 'Commentary: Somatic Cell Nuclear Transfer—Progress and Promise', *Stem Cells*, 26 (2008), 494–5.

[16] For an overview, see Kathy O. Lui et al., 'Embryonic Stem Cells: Overcoming the Immunological Barriers to Cell Replacement Therapy', *Current Stem Cell Research and Therapy*, 4 (2009), 70–80.

(1) continuous administration of immunosuppressive drugs (these have, however, serious side-effects and can also be lethal);

(2) setting up stem cell banks with a wide range of stem cell lines, so that at least one line is likely to be compatible with the immune system of a given patient (this would, however, require a large number of embryonic stem cell lines[17]);

(3) generating 'universal donor lines' which can be genetically modified to suit the immune system of a specific patient (however, this has been said to make such cells clinically unusable[18]);

(4) co-transplanting haematopoietic stem cells, which are immunologically naïve, with the embryonic stem cell-derived tissue to induce lifelong tolerance to the graft;[19] and

(5) combining embryonic stem cell technology with somatic cell nuclear transfer (SCNT) or cloning to generate replacement cells that are genetically identical to the patient.

The latter solution has attracted most attention in the ethical debate surrounding embryonic stem cell research. I return to this possibility in more detail in section 2.1.

It is, of course, possible that another solution will be found that has all the advantages, but none of the presumed *dis*advantages of embryonic stem cell research. The most obvious candidate is the induced pluripotent stem cell (iPSC) technique, which involves the direct reprogramming of somatic (body) cells to a pluripotent state using genetic manipulation. Just like embryonic stem cell research combined with SCNT, the iPSC technique allows the generation of customized pluripotent stem cells, for example, pluripotent stem cells genetically identical to a patient. However, the iPSC technique does not involve the creation or destruction of early embryos, thus avoiding the ethical problems associated with embryonic stem cell research. Some have argued that iPSC research could offer an ethically unproblematic replacement for embryonic stem cell research, thus obviating the need to continue embryonic stem cell research. However, as I will argue in more detail in section 4.4,

---

[17] Craig J. Taylor et al., 'Banking on Human Embryonic Stem Cells: Estimating the Number of Donor Cell Lines Needed for HLA Matching', *The Lancet*, 366 (2005), 2019–25.

[18] Cervera and Stojkovic, 'Commentary: Somatic Cell Nuclear Transfer'.

[19] Georg F. Beilhack et al., 'Purified Allogeneic Hematopoietic Stem Cell Transplantation Blocks Diabetes Pathogenesis in NOD Mice', *Diabetes*, 52 (2003), 59–68.

this conclusion is too quick, and this for two reasons. First, scientific evidence suggests that iPSCs and embryonic stem cells are different in important respects and that their respective benefits complement one another. Thus, the intended research and therapeutic goals of stem cell research can be best achieved by using both types of cells.[20] Second, I suggest it is a mistake to think that iPSC research, *as it is currently done*, completely avoids the ethical problems associated with embryonic stem cell research. Both types of research are so closely intertwined that iPSC research cannot be completely dissociated from embryonic stem cell research and thus from embryo destruction. Indeed, one could argue that iPSC research, as it is currently done, indirectly encourages embryo destruction.

What is important for now is that, despite some disadvantages, the special characteristics of embryonic stem cells make them better suited than adult stem cells and iPSCs for achieving certain important therapeutic and research aims. Thus, the case for embryonic stem cell research is strong. Embryonic stem cells are easy to obtain, available in large numbers, and can differentiate into virtually any kind of body cell. This is not to say that other types of stem cell are not useful. Adult stem cells, for example, have considerable advantages too and will no doubt be more suitable than embryonic stem cells for particular purposes (for example, haematopoietic stem cells for treating leukaemia and other blood disorders, and mesenchymal stem cells for treating osteoporosis and arthritis[21]). But most stem cell researchers, including those working with other types of stem cell, agree that research on embryonic stem cells is needed if we want to achieve all the intended goals of stem cell research.[22] Thus, abstaining from embryonic stem cell research will very likely result in avoidable deaths and suffering. The same moral reasons that count strongly in favour of stem cell research—reasons of

[20] Daisy A. Robinton and George Q. Daley, 'The Promise of Induced Pluripotent Stem Cells in Research and Therapy', *Nature*, 481 (2012), 295–305, 300.

[21] Ignazio Barbagallo et al., 'Overexpression of Heme Oxygenase-1 Increases Human Osteoblast Stem Cell Differentiation', *Journal of Bone and Mineral Metabolism*, 28 (2010), 276–88. Jennifer S. Park et al., 'The Effect of Matrix Stiffness on the Differentiation of Mesenchymal Stem Cells in Response to TGF- b', *Biomaterials*, 32 (2011), 3921–30.

[22] Giuseppe Testa, Lodovica Borghese, Julius A. Steinbeck, and Oliver Brüstle, 'Breakdown of the Potentiality Principle and its Impact on Global Stem Cell Research', *Cell Stem Cell*, 1 (2007), 153–6.

beneficence—count strongly in favour of *embryonic* stem cell research in particular.

Let us now consider the second question. What reasons, if any, are there to oppose embryonic stem cell research and, consequently, to forego its potential benefits?

1.3. Reasons for Opposing Embryonic Stem Cell Research

Destroying embryos

The derivation of embryonic stem cells currently involves the destruction of the early embryo's structure, thereby impeding its further development. (I will discuss proposed methods to derive embryonic stem cells without destroying the embryo in Chapter 4.) For those who hold the view that the early embryo is merely a lump of cells, embryonic stem cell research is comparable to research using any other type of body cell or tissue. However, for those who accord a significant moral status to the early embryo, the destruction of the embryo provides a strong moral reason to oppose embryonic stem cell research, sometimes a decisive reason.

I have not specified yet what I mean by 'significant moral status'. I use this to mean either a full moral status, or a high intermediate moral status that would normally rule out the deliberate destruction of embryos. Let me briefly clarify these views on the moral status of the embryo.

The full moral status view

Proponents of what I will refer to as 'the full moral status view' hold that the early embryo has the same moral status, that is, the same set of basic moral rights, claims, or interests as an ordinary adult human being. This view is sometimes expressed by saying that the early embryo is a person. In the debate about moral status, the term 'person' is typically used in a moral way, as shorthand for 'a being with full moral status'.[23]

---

[23] See e.g. Carson Strong, 'The Moral Status of Preembryos, Embryos, Foetuses, and Infants', *Journal of Medicine and Philosophy*, 22 (1997), 457–78.

Defenders of the full moral status view believe that the embryo acquires a full moral status, or personhood, from the moment of fertilization or an equivalent event such as the completion of SCNT, where a somatic cell is fused with an enucleated oocyte (see section 2.1 for technical details). One of the most ardent defenders of the full moral status view is the Roman Catholic Church. Its official view on this matter is formulated in *Dignitas Personae*:

The human being is to be respected and treated as a person from the moment of conception; and therefore from that same moment his rights as a person must be recognized, among which in the first place is the inviolable right of every innocent human being to life (n. 4).[24]

The full moral status view is not only common among Roman Catholics; it is also adopted by many Eastern Orthodox Christians, Evangelical Protestants, and other pro-life groups. Some states officially defend the full moral status view. Ireland, for example, protects the right to life of the unborn in its constitution. (Though it is unclear whether 'the unborn' includes early embryos.)

Because it is not my aim in this book to defend a particular view on the moral status of the embryo, I restrict myself here to briefly mentioning the two most popular arguments in defence of the full moral status view, and the most common objections to these arguments.

A first argument in support of the full moral status view is that an early embryo is a human being, and that all human beings have full moral status in virtue of their being human. An embryo should not be deliberately destroyed in research simply because it is human. This popular argument has been challenged for being 'speciecist', as it is not clear why belonging to a certain species has moral significance.[25] The fact that the embryo is human simply seems a criterion too arbitrary to have moral relevance for tracking moral status, just like belonging to a certain race or sex is too arbitrary to determine moral status. Another popular argument in support of the full moral status view is that an embryo, from the

---

[24] Pope John Paul II's *Evangelium Vitae* encyclical (1995), with reference to the *Donum Vitae*, and updated in *Dignitas Personae* (2008 n. 4) instruction of the Congregation for the Doctrine of Faith (1987).

[25] See e.g. Helga Kuhse and Peter Singer, 'Individuals, Humans, and Persons: the Issue of Moral Status', in Peter Singer and Helga Kuhse (eds), *Unsanctifying Human Life: Essays on Ethics* (Oxford: Wiley-Blackwell, 2002), 188–98.

moment of conception or an equivalent process, has the potential to develop into a being that is clearly a person and, therefore, should be protected as if it already were one. Many bioethicists and others have pointed out weaknesses in this 'potentiality argument'. An initial problem is one of logic: acorns are not oak trees, nor are eggs chickens or omelettes. Just because something has the potential to become something different, it does not follow that we should treat it as if it had already realized that potential. Unless and until we achieve immortality, all of us share one important and inexorable potential: we are all potentially dead—but it does not follow that we must be treated as though we are already dead.[26] Another problem with the potentiality argument is its scope. If the human embryo has the potential to become a human being and is supposedly morally important in virtue of that potential, then every other cell or group of cells with the same potential must be assigned equal moral status. This has been referred to as 'the extension argument'.[27] I will discuss it in more detail in section 3.2.

For many who hold the full moral status view, the fact that embryonic stem cell research relies on embryo destruction provides a decisive reason to oppose such research, regardless of how large its expected benefits are. For example John Meyer, a priest of the Opus Dei prelature, writes that 'the medical benefits which might accrue for some patients do not outweigh the grave consequences for the embryo that is killed in order to procure ES [embryonic stem] cells for medical therapy'.[28] Indeed, if the early embryo has the same basic claims, interests, or rights as a person, and one thinks that persons should not be killed for research purposes, however important these are, it follows that embryos too should not be killed in research, even if this could save many people's lives. Note that the term 'outweigh' in the quote may be somewhat misleading. Many who accord a full moral status to the embryo think that the embryo's right to life cannot be put in a scale, precisely *because* it is a (fundamental) right. It cannot be outweighed by countervailing considerations.

---

[26] Katrien Devolder and John Harris, 'The Ambiguity of the Embryo: Ethical Inconsistency in the Human Embryonic Stem Cell Debate', *Metaphilosophy*, 28/2–3 (2007), 153–69.

[27] David. B. Annis, 'Abortion and the Potentiality Principle', *Southern Journal of Philosophy*, 22 (1984), 155–63.

[28] John R. Meyer, 'Human Embryonic Stem Cells and Respect for Life', *Journal of Medical Ethics*, 26 (2000), 166–70.

Many of those who hold the full moral status view may nevertheless feel confronted with the Problem as they are faced with two conflicting values whose realization they find extremely important. Even if they believe that embryonic stem cell research is impermissible because it relies on, or involves embryo destruction, they also accept that it could significantly benefit a large number of people and that this provides a strong moral reason in favour of pursuing embryonic stem cell research. This moral reason can but does not need to be understood in consequentialist terms. It can, for example, also be understood in terms of duties, such as the duty to help those suffering from diseases and disabilities.

Thus, even though those who believe the embryo is a person may have no doubts that embryonic stem cell research is impermissible, they may at the same time strongly wish that the intended research goals of embryonic stem cell research will be achieved. This is nicely illustrated by the following quotation from an article written by ten authors holding the full moral status view:

> [W]e are all too aware of the massive destruction of human life in the womb through direct abortion as well as the creation and destruction of human embryos as a byproduct of new reproductive technologies. Pope John Paul II . . . was correct in describing us as a 'Culture of Death.' On the other hand, there is a strong vein in the Catholic tradition supporting those who defend the stewardship that men and women enjoy because they are made in the image and likeness of God. Our human dignity and, indeed, mandate from the Creator, is to try to discover the many remarkable sources of healing and alleviation of suffering that are present right in our very created beings. Such is the challenge of modern genetic and cell research. The question is, how can stem cell research be done while still respecting human life at the same time?[29]

Thus, even if one believes embryonic stem cell research is impermissible, one might nevertheless feel an urgent need to find a solution to the Problem.

The intermediate moral status view

Many are not convinced by the arguments advanced in support of the full moral status view. They may also think that this view has implausible

---

[29] Michael R. Prieur et al., 'Stem Cell Research in a Catholic Institution: Yes or No?', *Kennedy Institute of Ethics Journal*, 16 (2006), 73–98, 84.

implications, for example, in so-called 'embryo rescue cases'.[30] Suppose that a thousand embryos have been created in the context of IVF treatments, and that these embryos are no longer wanted for reproductive purposes. They are being kept frozen in a nitrogen freezer in a warehouse. One day a fire breaks out in the warehouse. Not only the embryos' lives are at stake, but also that of an employee at the warehouse. As a fire fighter you are faced with a choice: either you can drag the freezer outside to rescue the embryos, or you can rescue the employee. You cannot do both. Intuitively it seems clear that you should rescue the employee, but if embryos have full moral status then you should save the embryos as it generally considered to be better to save thousands persons instead of one. It thus seems that the full moral status view is incompatible with commonly held intuitions. It may also have implausible implications in real-life cases. If embryos are persons, then we should, for example, exert great efforts to prevent spontaneous abortion as this would be one of the greatest problems of our time. It has been estimated that spontaneous abortion kills thirty times more people (if embryos and foetuses are people) than cancer does. However, it seems implausible that we should prioritize the prevention of spontaneous abortion over the prevention and treatment of cancer. Thus, the view that embryos are persons seems incompatible with our views about the importance of spontaneous abortion.[31]

Some of those who disagree with the full moral status view nevertheless think that the embryo has at least some intrinsic value, that is, some value in and of itself, regardless of its instrumental value or usefulness. They accord the embryo an intermediate moral status—a moral status somewhere in between that of a person and that of an ordinary body cell. They may believe that this intermediate moral status gradually increases during pregnancy—and perhaps infancy—until full moral status is attained, or they may think that there is some threshold, or a set of thresholds, at which moral status increases until full moral status is acquired.

[30] See e.g. Matthew S. Liao, 'The Embryo Rescue Case', *Theoretical Medicine and Bioethics*, 27 (2006), 141–7. George J. Annas, 'A French Homunculus in a Tennessee Court', *Hastings Center Report*, 19 (1989), 20–2.

[31] Leonard M. Fleck, 'Abortion, Deformed Fetuses, and the Omega Pill', *Philosophical Studies*, 36 (1979), 271–83. Toby Ord, 'The Scourge: Moral Implications of Natural Embryo Loss', *American Journal of Bioethics*, 8 (2008), 12–19.

The two main arguments in defence of the intermediate moral status view are similar to those adduced in defence of the full moral status view: although the embryo does not have the same rights as an ordinary adult human being, it has an intrinsic value in virtue either of being human, or of having the potential to become a being that is clearly a person.

According to the intermediate moral status view, deliberately destroying embryos is always *pro tanto* wrong, which means that there is some factor that militates in favour of its wrongness, though this could be outweighed by countervailing considerations, such as the fact that destroying an embryo would produce great benefits of a certain kind. To better understand this view it is useful to refer to the moral status accorded to certain animals. Many people accord an intermediate moral status to monkeys. If monkeys have an intermediate moral status then there are moral reasons not to deliberately kill them. This reason can, however, be outweighed by other reasons. Killing monkeys in medical experiments may be justified if this will prevent significant harm to many people. However, the development of cosmetics may not provide a sufficient reason to outweigh the deliberate killing of monkeys. Whether one thinks it does will depend on precisely what intermediate moral status one accords to monkeys and how important one thinks the development of cosmetics is. Likewise, whether one thinks that reasons of beneficence in favour of embryonic stem cell research outweigh the destruction of embryos will depend on precisely what intermediate moral status one accords to the embryo and on how large the expected benefits of embryonic stem cell research are. Some who hold the intermediate moral status view have argued that alternative types of stem cell research, like research with adult stem cells, should be explored first and that embryonic stem cell research should be considered only if and when it becomes clear that adult stem cell research fails to achieve the desired research goals. Others concede that some embryonic stem cell research may be done if scientists can present convincing arguments for the necessity of such research to achieve important therapeutic and research goals efficiently. The problem with the latter view is that many of the facts about the benefits of stem cell research are not presently known and that these uncertainties will not be resolved if certain types of research cannot be done because of prohibitive or restrictive regulations. This is the catch-22 for scientists who want to prove the promising potential of embryonic stem cell research. As mentioned earlier, whether the expected benefits of embryonic stem cell research outweigh the costs to the embryo will also partly depend on exactly how high the intermediate moral status is that one accords to the embryo, as this could be anything from somewhat above the moral status of a liver cell to just below a full moral status. Obviously, the higher the intermediate moral status one accords to the embryo the stronger the countervailing reasons have to be for research involving embryo destruction to be permissible.

For some holding the intermediate moral status view the Problem does not arise. They find that the expected benefits of embryonic stem cell research clearly provide a sufficiently strong reason to accept the research, even if this involves embryo destruction, since the intermediate moral status that they accord to the embryo is rather low. They do not find it problematic that early embryos are destroyed if this can benefit people. However, for those who accord a high intermediate moral status to the embryo—one much closer to that of a person—the fact that embryos are destroyed in embryonic stem cell research may provide a strong reason against such research, perhaps even a reason that outweighs reasons for conducting the research. Like many who accord a full moral status to the embryo, they experience the Problem as very real, since they deeply care about protecting embryos as well as about the wellbeing of patients suffering from currently incurable diseases who could be helped thanks to embryonic stem cell research. Some may think that the potential benefits of the research outweigh the loss of the embryos' lives, others may think they do not, or be indecisive. In any case, for many according a high intermediate moral status to the embryo, the Problem is real and resolving it is not only desirable, but urgent.

It is not my aim in this book to defend a particular view on the moral status of the embryo, though my arguments will put some such views under pressure. Throughout this book, I will be assuming that the embryo has a significant moral status, that is, a full moral status or a somewhat lower moral status than that but one that is nevertheless significant. This is because I wish to meet those who are confronted with the Problem on their own ground. People are extremely reluctant to modify their strongly and deeply held views on the moral status of the early embryo, even in light of strong arguments. My approach will therefore be to investigate the coherence of the main ethical positions on embryonic stem cell research, taking their assumptions about moral status as a fixed point. I touch upon the underlying justifications for views on moral status only insofar as this is relevant to my analysis of the responses to the Problem.

1.4. Two Types of Response to the Problem

The view that the embryo has a significant moral status has of course been challenged before, for example in the contexts of abortion, the use of contraception, and assisted reproduction. Some therefore conclude that the embryonic stem cell debate is not all that interesting as it does not raise new ethical issues. However, I think they are mistaken. The fact that the embryonic stem cell debate reignites 'old' ethical issues about the moral status of the embryo is exactly what makes it so interesting.

Every justification for an ethical stance on embryonic stem cell research inevitably touches upon earlier justifications of views about related practices where the protection of the embryo or foetus is at stake, such as abortion, assisted reproduction, and the use of contraceptives. This is also true at the level of policymaking where every justification of embryonic stem cell policy touches upon earlier justifications of policies in these related contexts. However, the important difference between embryonic stem cell research and practices like abortion or IVF is that a much larger section of society has an interest in it, as we and our loved ones are all potential patients who may one day benefit from the fruits of embryonic stem cell research. This has had remarkable consequences for the course the stem cell debate has taken and, subsequently, for stem cell policymaking. This is well captured by the following extract of a speech by US senator Bill Frist—a fervent opponent of abortion and IVF:

If your daughter has diabetes, if your father has Parkinson's, if your sister has a spinal cord injury, your views will be swayed more powerfully than you can imagine by the hope that cure will be found in those magnificent cells, recently discovered, that today originate only in an embryo.[32]

The difficulty for conservatives like Frist is to reconcile reasons *for* embryonic stem cell research with pro-life views on the protection of

---

[32] Bill Frist, *A Senator Speaks Out on Ethics, Respect, and Compassion* (Washington, DC: Monument Press, 2005), 235.

the embryo in the context of IVF, abortion, and so forth. If one rejects the destruction of embryos for particular beneficial purposes, how can one justify tolerating, or even supporting the destruction of embryos for other, seemingly morally equivalent purposes?[33]

Tension between the desire to reap the benefits of embryonic stem cell research and concerns about destroying embryos is also found at the level of public policymaking. For example, some countries with restrictive regulations regarding the protection of the embryo in the context of IVF, such as Germany and Italy, allow at least some embryonic stem cell research. Here too, the difficulty is to allow such research without violating the spirit of existing regulations regarding other practices where the protection of the embryo is at stake. However, in this book, I focus on *ethical* positions—views about which practices are ethically acceptable and which are ethically unacceptable—not policies (though, of course, the ethical positions discussed have influenced policies). Only in Chapter 5 do I discuss some implications of my conclusions regarding these ethical positions for stem cell policies.

One way to find a more consistent ethical position for those who are confronted with the Problem would be to simply accord a lower moral status to the embryo, one that would allow embryo destruction to be (more easily) outweighed by the expected benefits of embryonic stem cell research, as well as by important benefits in the context of abortion and perhaps IVF. However, people are extremely reluctant to give up on their views about the moral status of the embryo and the course the embryonic stem cell debate has taken has reconfirmed this. Those who accord a significant moral status to the embryo have tried very hard to find other ways to resolve the Problem, ways that do not require giving up the view that the embryo has a significant moral status. A first type of response has been to adopt a middle-ground position, that is, a position between the dominant opposing views on the permissibility of embryonic stem cell research. Such a position defends limited embryonic stem

---

[33] I am not saying that it is necessarily inconsistent to defend embryo destruction in one context but not in another. What I am saying is that any attempt to explain a presumed moral difference between embryo destruction in various contexts is likely to put the view that the embryo has a significant moral status under pressure. For a defence of the view that one can defend abortion without being committed to defend embryonic stem cell research, see Elizabeth Harman, 'How is the Ethics of Stem Cell Research Different from the Ethics of Abortion?', *Metaphilosophy*, 38 (2007), 207–25.

cell research, that is, certain types or aspects of embryonic stem cell research. The two main middle-ground positions in the embryonic stem cell debate are (i) the 'discarded–created distinction', which accepts the destruction of embryos donated to scientific research by couples undergoing IVF but rejects the creation and destruction of embryos created especially for the purpose of research, and (ii) the 'use–derivation distinction', which accepts the use but not the derivation of embryonic stem cells. A second type of response to the Problem has been to develop or defend technical solutions to the ethical issues raised by embryonic stem cell research. A number of techniques have been proposed to obtain embryonic stem cells, or their functional equivalents, that do not involve harming or destroying embryos. The most important of these techniques is the induced pluripotent stem cell technique, but other techniques have been proposed.

My view is that both types of response to the Problem, as they have been formulated to date, face serious shortcomings as correct ethical positions and fail to fully solve the Problem. My aim in this book is to defend this view.

1.5. The Plan

I have now introduced the Problem and the two main types of response to it. In the remaining chapters, I examine the arguments that have been advanced in defence of these responses.

Chapters 2 and 3 focus on the first type of response: defending a middle-ground position. In Chapter 2, I discuss the discarded–created distinction. This position holds that it may be permissible to use and derive stem cells from surplus embryos created in the context of fertility treatments and donated for research, but that it is always impermissible to use and derive stem cells from embryos created especially for the purpose of research. I argue that there is a presumption against this position, as in both types of research the expected benefits and moral costs seem so similar that either the costs should outweigh the benefits in *both* cases or in *neither* case. I then investigate whether any of the arguments adduced in support of the discarded–created distinction can override this presumption. I discuss arguments that appeal to the nothing-is-lost principle, the doctrine of double effect, and the notion of respect.

Chapter 3 focuses on the use–derivation distinction. This middle-ground position holds that it may be permissible to *use* embryonic stem cells in research but that it is always impermissible to *derive* embryonic stem cells, as this process involves embryo destruction. I first investigate an assumption underlying this position, namely that embryonic stem cells are neither embryos nor their moral equivalents. I then turn to consider the main claim offered in support of the use–derivation distinction: that using embryonic stem cells does not encourage embryo destruction in a way that makes it presumptively wrong. I focus on two questions. Does a researcher, by merely using embryonic stem cells, increase the total number of embryos destroyed in the context of stem cell research? And, if a researcher does *not* increase the number of embryos destroyed, is this sufficient to show that using embryonic stem cells does not encourage embryo destruction in a way that makes it presumptively wrong?

In Chapter 4, I address the second type of response to the Problem: offering a technical solution. I discuss the various ways in which it has been suggested that we might obtain embryonic stem cells, or their functional equivalents, without harming embryos. These include the use of organismically dead embryos, blastomere biopsy, the blastocyst transfer method, altered nuclear transfer, and parthenogenesis. The main question is whether these techniques really avoid the problem of embryo destruction while enabling us to achieve the intended goals of stem cell research. I then discuss induced pluripotent stem cell research. It has been claimed that this research is the most promising alternative to embryonic stem cell research and even marks the end of the embryonic stem cell debate. I will challenge this claim.

Finally, in Chapter 5, I briefly summarize my findings and mention a seemingly shocking implication of these findings, together with a possible strategy for avoiding this implication. I also deal with an important question that I ignore in the preceding chapters: should we accept or defend any of the views considered in the earlier chapters not as correct ethical positions but as compromise positions?

2

The Discarded–Created Distinction

2.1. The Discarded–Created Distinction

Recall:

> *The Problem.* Either one supports embryonic stem cell research and accepts the resulting embryo destruction, or one opposes embryonic stem cell research and accepts that its potential benefits will be foregone.

As mentioned in Chapter 1, the Problem only exists for those who accord a significant moral status to the embryo—a full moral status or a high intermediate moral status—and who believe that the fact that embryonic stem cell research involves embryo destruction provides a strong or even a decisive moral reason against such research.

Since people are generally reluctant to modify their deeply held views on the moral status of the embryo, many have looked for other ways to solve or circumvent the Problem. A popular strategy has been to adopt a middle-ground position, that is, an ethical position between the dominant opposing views on the permissibility of embryonic stem cell research. These opposing views hold respectively that all embryonic stem cell research is morally unacceptable and that embryonic stem cell research is no more problematic than other kinds of research in cell biology. The aim of these middle-ground positions has been to accept as many types or aspects of embryonic stem cell research as is compatible with the view that the embryo has a significant moral status. One middle-ground position that has been widely defended and that has served as an ethical basis for stem cell policy in many Western countries is

The Discarded-Created Distinction.[1] It is presumptively permissible to derive and use stem cells from embryos discarded following in vitro fertilization (IVF). However, it is impermissible to derive and use stem cells from embryos created solely for the purpose of stem cell research or therapy.

The discarded–created distinction draws a moral line between two types of embryonic stem cell research based on the origin of the embryos used to derive stem cells: embryos discarded following IVF and embryos created especially for the purpose of stem cell research.[2]

Discarded embryos

The great majority of currently existing embryonic stem cell lines originate from embryos discarded following IVF. A woman undergoing IVF receives hormone therapy to stimulate the development and maturation of multiple oocytes (eggs). After retrieval, the oocytes are fertilized with semen in culture media. In most countries where IVF is practised, on average five to ten embryos are produced, one or two of which are transferred to the woman's uterus in an attempt to initiate a pregnancy. The remaining embryos are cryopreserved in nitrogen freezers. If an attempt to achieve a pregnancy fails, one or two embryos can be thawed for another attempt. The cryopreservation of several embryos has the advantage that it reduces the risk of twin or triplet pregnancies. One can implant one embryo per attempt. If an attempt fails, one can simply thaw another embryo and try again. Another (related) major advantage of this way of doing IVF is that the woman does not have to undergo the hormone therapy and egg retrieval procedure, which entail some risk and discomfort, before each attempt to generate a pregnancy. Though some hormones need to be administered to prepare the endometrium for implantation, it is not necessary to administer additional hormones to stimulate the ovaries.

---

[1] I borrow the term 'discarded–created distinction' from the National Advisory Bioethics Commission's report *Ethical Issues in Human Stem Cell Research*, 55.

[2] See e.g. *The 'Warnock Report'*, Report of the Committee of Inquiry into Human Fertilisation and Embryology (London: Her Majesty's Stationery Office, 1978). See also the National Institutes of Health, Ad Hoc Group of Consultants to the Advisory Committee to the Director, *Report of the Human Embryo Research Panel* (Washington, DC: NIH, 1994). Note that the discarded–created distinction is not new to the stem cell debate. It has been defended in the context of embryo research in general.

Typically individuals or couples embarking on an IVF treatment must indicate one of the following three options for handling of any surplus embryos, that is, embryos no longer wanted by the individual or couple, usually because their wish for a child has been fulfilled: (1) anonymous donation to other infertile couples, (2) donation to scientific research, or (3) letting the embryos perish. Note that the two last options both involve destruction of the embryo, and thus prevent it from developing into a child. The great majority of existing embryonic stem cell lines has been obtained from surplus IVF embryos donated for research—as under option (2). I will refer to such embryos as *discarded embryos*.

Research embryos

There is an alternative source of embryonic stem cells. Embryonic stem cells could also be derived from embryos especially created for the purpose of research. I will refer to such embryos as *research embryos*. The term 'created' in the 'discarded–created distinction' may be somewhat confusing as IVF embryos have, of course, also been created, just for a different purpose. The relevant difference is that discarded embryos were created for reproductive purposes, whereas research embryos were created solely for the purpose of research. I hope that the term 'discarded–created distinction' will nevertheless become somewhat familiar as this chapter proceeds.

Research embryos could be generated in the laboratory by fertilizing donor oocytes with donor sperm. This involves the application of IVF not to generate a pregnancy but to produce embryos that could be used as a source of stem cells. Research embryos could also be produced through other techniques, including through parthenogenesis (a form of asexual reproduction in which oocytes can develop into embryos without being fertilized by sperm—I discuss this technique in section 4.3) and, more important for now, through cloning. In the context of stem cell research, cloning would not be used to create offspring, but to generate customized embryonic stem cells, for example, stem cells that are genetically identical to the patient. The technique, known as somatic cell nuclear transfer (SCNT), involves transferring the nucleus of a somatic (body) cell into an oocyte from which the nucleus and thus most of the DNA has been removed.[3] The enucleated oocyte is then

---

[3] The oocyte will still contain mitochondrial DNA, which resides in the cytoplasm outside of the cell nucleus.

treated with an electric current in order to stimulate cell division, resulting in the formation of an embryo. The embryo is a clone of, and thus virtually genetically identical to, the donor of the somatic cell, say a patient. Stem cells derived from the embryo would thus also be genetically identical to the patient.[4]

That embryonic stem cells, and their derivatives, would be genetically identical to the patient has significant advantages. They would be a better match to the patient's immune system than embryonic stem cells originating from discarded embryos. As mentioned in Chapter 1, one of the major problems in transplantation medicine is the rejection of the transplanted material by the immune system, or the reverse. Such immunorejection could be prevented by lifelong treatment with immunosuppressive drugs, but these have serious side-effects and can be lethal. Therapies using stem cells from embryos created via SCNT (henceforth just 'SCNT embryos') may help overcome the problem of immunorejection, reducing the need for long-term use of immunosuppressants. Though such therapies are not yet on the horizon for humans, scientists have provided proof of concept for them in the mouse. For example, in 2002, a research team at the Harvard Stem Cell Institute created a mouse with a mouse variant of Severe Combined Immunodeficiency Disease (commonly known as the 'boy in the bubble disease' when it occurs in humans). They took cells from the mouse's tail, subjected these to the cloning process, produced embryonic stem cells derived from the cloned mice embryos, introduced genes into these embryonic stem cells to correct the genetic defect, and reintroduced the cells into the mouse, curing the disease.[5]

A more immediate application of SCNT would be to create customized embryonic stem cells for biomedical research, including for drug discovery and toxicity testing.[6] Customized embryonic stem cells could provide unique tools to generate *in vitro* models to study genetic disease.

---

[4] The stem cells may not be completely genetically identical to the patient. This is because the mitochondrial DNA will typically come from an oocyte donor. If the patient is a woman she could, in principle, be the donor of the somatic cell *and* the oocyte. In that case, the stem cells, and their derivatives would be genetically identical to the patient.

[5] William M. Rideout et al., 'Correction of a Genetic Defect by Nuclear Transplantation and Combined Cell and Gene Therapy', *Cell*, 109 (2002), 17–27.

[6] Rita Pilar Cervera and Miodrag Stojkovic, 'Commentary: Somatic Cell Nuclear Transfer—Progress and Promise', *Stem Cells*, 26 (2008), 494–5.

Researchers could create large numbers of embryonic stem cells genetically identical to the patient and then experiment on these in order to understand the particular features of the disease in that person. For example, they could coax the embryonic stem cells to differentiate into different cell types and monitor the progress of the disease as it develops inside these cells. This would allow the investigation of the early, presymptomatic phases of the disease, which are otherwise difficult to access, as well as the study of genetic predispositions, and other contributing factors to the disease, whether genetic, epigenetic, or environmental. Furthermore, these cells could be used to test potential treatments. They could, for example, be used to test candidate drug therapies to predict their likely toxicity. This would avoid dangerous exposure of the patient to sometimes highly experimental drugs.

Thus, research using SCNT embryos holds the potential to achieve research and therapeutic goals that would be much more difficult or perhaps impossible to achieve using embryonic stem cells from discarded embryos, as these are not normally genetically identical to the patient.[7] At this point one could point out that, even though it is true that the same therapeutic and research goals cannot be achieved using discarded embryos, a more recent development—induced pluripotent stem cell (iPSC) research—could achieve these goals, making the application of SCNT in stem cell research obsolete.[8] However, as I will argue in section 4.4, iPSC research is unlikely to make SCNT research obsolete. Thus, it remains true that, at the moment, research using SCNT embryos could achieve therapeutic and research goals that we are unlikely to achieve through other means.

Research into SCNT in humans is in its infancy. At the time of writing, researchers still have to learn how to routinely produce SCNT embryos and how to derive stem cells from them. One of the main problems is that such research requires a large supply of good-quality oocytes. As mentioned earlier, the oocyte retrieval procedure is not without risk and discomfort. As a result, few women volunteer to donate their oocytes to

---

[7] Some of the research could be done using embryos discarded following IVF combined with preimplantation genetic diagnosis. However, there are some disadvantages to using these embryos. See e.g. Yuri Verlinsky et al., 'Preimplantation Diagnosis for Immunodeficiencies', *Reproductive BioMedicine Online*, 14 (2007), 214–23.

[8] Jose B. Cibelli, 'Is Therapeutic Cloning Dead?', *Science*, 318 (2007), 1879–80.

stem cell research. Allowing a market for oocytes may increase the number of oocytes available for research, but because of ethical concerns regarding exploitation of women and commodification of body materials, most countries do not allow such a market. The shortage of donor oocytes has led scientists to look for alternatives, such as the use of animal oocytes, oocytes derived from existing stem-cell lines, or oocytes obtained through the maturation of germ cells from the ovaries of aborted foetuses. Somatic cells have also been reprogrammed to a pluripotent state after fusion with embryonic stem cells, instead of with oocytes.[9] Another reason why research using SCNT embryos is in its infancy is because such embryos would be *research embryos* and thus, according to the discarded–created distinction, it would be impermissible to derive and use stem cells from them. As many countries have based their stem cell regulations on the discarded–created distinction, research into SCNT embryos has been prohibited or severely restricted in most countries.

The obvious question that arises is how it can be permissible to destroy discarded embryos for stem cell research but not research embryos. Why is the destruction of research embryos to obtain stem cells worse, from a moral point of view, than the destruction of discarded embryos, and to such an extent that the latter is presumptively ethically permissible but the former not? In the remainder of this chapter, I try to find a satisfactory answer to this question.

I start by investigating how proponents of the discarded–created distinction justify the destruction of discarded embryos to obtain stem cells. I show that the justification for destroying discarded embryos also applies, at least at first sight, to the destruction of research embryos. This suggests that there should be a presumption against the discarded–created distinction. I then consider whether this presumption can be overridden. After exploring the main arguments in support of the discarded–created distinction, I conclude that none of these arguments hold and that, until better arguments are offered, we should reject the discarded–created distinction as a solid ethical position.

---

[9] Chad A. Cowan, Jocelyn Atienza, Douglas A. Melton, and Kevin Eggan, 'Nuclear Reprogramming of Somatic Cells After Fusion with Human Embryonic Stem Cells', *Science*, 309 (2005), 1369–73.

First, let us consider how proponents of the discarded–created distinction justify the destruction of discarded embryos. Remember that we are assuming throughout that the embryo has a significant moral status: a full moral status, or a high intermediate moral status.

2.2. Justifying the Destruction of Discarded Embryos

Beneficence

As outlined in Chapter 1, there are strong reasons of beneficence to pursue embryonic stem cell research. Everyone could potentially benefit from the fruits of such research. It could help us to prevent and treat a wide range of diseases and disabilities, including devastating ones for which we currently do not have a treatment and which result in imminent death or an extremely low quality of life. Failing to pursue embryonic stem cell research can be expected to result in many avoidable premature deaths and much avoidable suffering.

Defenders of the discarded–created distinction have appealed to reasons of beneficence to justify destroying discarded embryos to obtain stem cells.[10] For example, in its 1999 report *Ethical Issues in Human Stem Cell Research*, the US National Bioethics Advisory Commission (NBAC) wrote that the ban on federal funding for research that involves harming or destroying embryos

conflicts with several of the ethical goals of medicine, especially healing, prevention, and research—goals that are rightly characterized by the principles of beneficence and non-maleficence, jointly encouraging the pursuit of each social benefit and avoiding or ameliorating potential harm.[11]

Proportionality

Even if one thinks that reasons of beneficence are strong reasons for pursuing research on discarded embryos one may of course argue that these reasons are not strong *enough* to outweigh the countervailing

---

[10] See e.g. Commission of the European Communities, *Commission Staff Working Paper: Report on Human Embryonic Stem Cell Research* (Brussels: Commission of the European Communities, 2003), 9.

[11] NBAC, *Ethical Issues*, 69.

reasons for not destroying embryos. Which reasons prevail will depend, at least in part, on how great the expected benefits of embryonic stem cell research are relative to the moral costs of embryo destruction. Proponents of the discarded–created distinction evidently believe that the expected benefits are large enough, relative to the costs, to justify the destruction of discarded embryos. This is sometimes made explicit. For example, the NBAC wrote that 'the potential benefits of the research outweigh the harms to the embryos that are destroyed in the research process'.[12]

The obvious question that arises, then, is the following. If the expected benefits of embryonic stem cell research using discarded embryos are sufficient to outweigh the moral costs of destroying discarded embryos, why do the expected benefits of research with research embryos not outweigh the moral costs of destroying research embryos?[13] It seems that, at first sight, the expected costs and benefits are so similar that either the costs should outweigh the benefits in both cases, or in neither case. The stem cell derivation procedure is the same in both types of research, and most would agree that the moral status of discarded embryos and research embryos is the same. (Indeed, those who disagree typically accord a *lower* moral status to research embryos than to discarded embryos as the former currently cannot give rise to live offspring.[14]) This suggests there should be a presumption against the discarded–created distinction. I now turn to consider how one might nevertheless defend the discarded–created distinction by appealing to arguments that override this presumption.

2.3. The Least Controversial Approach

One argument that could override the presumption against the discarded–created distinction is that, even if the benefits of embryonic stem cell research outweigh the destruction of both discarded embryos and research embryos, we should only use discarded embryos to obtain

---

[12] NBAC, *Ethical Issues*, 52.

[13] Note that moral costs could include a violation of a deontological rule. I am thus not restricting myself to a consequentialist approach here.

[14] See e.g. Paul R. McHugh, 'Zygote and "Clonote": The Ethical Use of Embryonic Stem Cells', *New England Journal of Medicine*, 351 (2004), 209–10.

stem cells because, if we have different ways of achieving our goals, we should always opt for the least controversial or the least offensive approach.[15] This argument, however, cannot convincingly justify the discarded–created distinction.

First, it is not true that we can achieve our research goals by using discarded embryos only. As mentioned earlier, some research and therapeutic goals can only be achieved using research embryos, especially those generated through SCNT, as these would allow us to produce customized embryonic stem cells. Second, determining what approach is the least controversial is, of course, controversial itself and will partly depend on who decides what is most controversial and on how well people are informed about the variety of issues raised by different types of stem cell research. It is not obvious why the embryo's moral status should be the only relevant or the most important consideration for determining how controversial certain types of stem cell research are. Other considerations that have received less attention in the stem cell debate may also need to be taken into account, including whether the use of alternative types of stem cells will slow down the research, what risks they involve to patients, what the economic cost will be, and so forth.[16] For example, obtaining neuronal stem cells from patients through brain biopsy does not involve embryo destruction but may pose a significant risk to the patient and may, therefore, be more controversial than using stem cells from research embryos. Moreover, as pointed out earlier, some think that SCNT embryos have lower moral status than discarded embryos and that it is therefore less controversial to use SCNT embryos to obtain stem cells than to use discarded embryos.

Stating that we should reject destructive research with research embryos simply because it is more controversial than research with discarded embryos not only assumes too quickly that both types of research will enable us to achieve the same research goals, but also begs the question. That research with research embryos is the most controversial approach is exactly what needs to be argued for.

[15] Joseph C. Fletcher, 'NBAC's Arguments on Embryo Research: Strengths and Weaknesses', in Suzanne Holland, Karen Lebacqz, and Laurie Zoloth (eds), *The Human Embryonic Stem Cell Debate: Science, Ethics, and Public Policy* (Cambridge, Mass.: MIT Press, 2001), 61–72.

[16] Guido Pennings and André Van Steirteghem, 'The Subsidiarity Principle in the Context of Embryonic Stem Cell Research', *Human Reproduction*, 19 (2004), 1060–4.

That leaves us with our initial question: why is it worse to destroy research embryos than to destroy discarded embryos to obtain stem cells?

2.4. Nothing-is-Lost

The nothing-is-lost principle

One popular and intuitively appealing argument in defence of the discarded–created distinction holds that destructive research on discarded embryos is presumptively permissible since these embryos are never going to be used for reproductive purposes even if not used in research. The thought is that destroying discarded embryos does not result in any loss that was not going to occur in any case. Gene Outka, for example, writes that

embryos in appreciable numbers have now been discarded or frozen in perpetuity. They will die, unimplanted, in any case. Nothing more will be lost by their becoming subjects of research.[17]

It is then argued that, because nothing is lost, and significant goods are expected to come out of research with discarded embryos, it is presumptively permissible to conduct such research, even if embryos have a significant moral status and it is therefore normally impermissible to conduct destructive research on them. It is further argued that an equivalent argument cannot justify destructive research on research embryos.[18]

In a similar vein, George Annas, Arthur Caplan, and Sherman Elias write that

Although the destruction of a human embryo is lamentable, there is a considerable moral difference between creating and destroying embryos solely to obtain stem cells and destroying unwanted human embryos that will never be used for reproductive purposes, to achieve benefit for those with serious diseases and disorders. The former involves the creation solely for the purpose of destruction whereas the latter involves salvaging something of value from a situation from which nothing else can be gained.[19]

---

[17] Gene Outka, 'The Ethics of Embryonic Stem Cell Research and the Principle of Nothing is Lost', *Yale Journal of Health Policy Law and Ethics*, 9 (2009), 596.

[18] Gene Outka, 'The Ethics of Human Stem Cell Research', *Kennedy Institute of Ethics Journal*, 12 (2002), 175–213. Michael R. Prieur et al., 'Stem Cell Research in a Catholic Institution: Yes or No?', *Kennedy Institute of Ethics Journal*, 16 (2006), 73–98.

[19] George J. Annas, Arthur Caplan, and Sherman Elias, 'Stem Cell Politics, Ethics and Medical Progress', *Nature Medicine*, 5 (1999), 1340.

The principle (often implicitly) appealed to in these arguments could be formulated as follows

The Nothing-is-Lost principle (NILp). It is presumptively permissible to intentionally cause a certain loss that it would normally be impermissible to intentionally cause if (1) the loss is going to occur in any case, and (2) something good is expected to come out of causing the loss.

Note that the application of NILp alone can only justify a *qualified* conclusion: that it is *presumptively* permissible to destroy discarded embryos. For the destruction of discarded embryos to be permissible, NILp should be correct, the conditions specified in NILp should be met, and there should be nothing that defeats the presumption that destroying discarded embryos is permissible. (For example, one consideration that would defeat this presumption is that no parental consent was obtained to destroy the embryo.)

In the next section, I do not focus on possible defeaters. Instead, I investigate whether it is true that NILp *presumptively* justifies destroying discarded embryos. If not, the principle cannot support the discarded-created distinction.[20]

I will first investigate whether the argument works, assuming the embryo has a full moral status. Though the majority of defenders of the discarded−created distinction do not ascribe a full moral status to the embryo, there are at least three reasons to consider whether the distinction could be sustained on this view:

(i) at least some people who defend the distinction hold the full moral status view,

(ii) examining the plausibility of the distinction on the assumption that the embryo has full moral status is a helpful strategy to better understand and critically examine the principles appealed to in the arguments, and

(iii) many who hold the full moral status view defend some weaker version of the discarded−created distinction. (For example, they only accept the use of embryonic stem cells from discarded embryos

---

[20] The section on the nothing-is-lost principle is based on Katrien Devolder, 'Killing Discarded Embryos and the Nothing-is-Lost Principle', *Journal of Applied Philosophy*, 30 (2013), 289–303.

but not from research embryos, thus drawing a moral distinction between the destruction of discarded and research embryos. In drawing this distinction, they, sometimes implicitly, appeal to arguments adduced in defence of the discarded–created distinction.[21])

Nothing-is-lost and the killing of persons

Suppose you like furniture made of tropical wood but agree that it is unethical to fell endangered trees to construct such furniture. One day you discover that an endangered tropical tree in your garden has a terminal disease. After careful consideration, you fell the tree to make a table out of it. Intuitively it seems correct that NILp could justify your action: though it is perhaps normally impermissible to fell endangered trees to construct furniture, the tree in your garden was going to die soon in any case, and something good—a beautiful table—comes out of your felling it.

But can NILp plausibly be appealed to if the loss that is going to occur in any case is the life of a being of significant moral status, perhaps that of a person? If not, it cannot justify destroying discarded embryos, on our assumption that these embryos have a significant moral status.

Consider this slightly modified version of Bernard Williams' famous *Jim and the Indians* case.[22]

> *Tim and the Indians.* Tim arrives in a South American town where twenty Indians are just about to be killed by a group of soldiers under the command of an army captain. The captain makes Tim an offer: if Tim kills one Indian, Mika, the others will be let off. If Tim refuses the offer, the captain will do what he would have done had Tim not arrived: have the soldiers kill all twenty Indians, including Mika. Tim wonders whether he could get hold of the gun and kill the captain and the soldiers, but it is clear that this is not going to work. Attempting this would result in all the Indians and himself being killed.

It is somewhat plausible that it may be permissible for Tim to kill Mika because (1) the loss is going to occur in any case (Mika is going to die

---

[21] See e.g. Prieur et al., 'Stem Cell Research in a Catholic Institution'.

[22] Bernard A. O. Williams, 'A Critique of Utilitarianism', in J. J. C. Smart and Bernard A. O. Williams (eds), *Utilitarianism: For and Against* (Cambridge: Cambridge University Press, 1973), 82–117. My change consists in specifying which Indian is going to be killed in any case.

regardless) and (2) something good is expected to come out of Tim causing the loss (the other Indians will be saved). So it is somewhat plausible that NILp could justify Tim killing Mika. (Note that Williams did not use *Jim and the Indians* to illustrate NILp. I borrow the case because a slightly modified version of it shows that NILp could plausibly justify killing a person.)

Nothing-is-lost and the destruction of discarded embryos

Since it is somewhat plausible that NILp could justify killing a person, it is not yet ruled out that it could justify destroying a discarded embryo. For the latter to be presumptively permissible, it will have to be true that (1) the loss is going to occur in any case, and (2) something good is expected to come out of causing the loss.

Defenders of the discarded–created distinction have argued that (1) and (2) are true. For example, according to Gene Outka,

> it is correct to view embryos in reproductive clinics who are bound either to be discarded or frozen in perpetuity as innocent lives who will die in any case, and those third parties with Alzheimer's, Parkinson's, and other diseases as other innocent lives who may be saved, or at least helped, by virtue of research on such embryos.[23]

That others will expectedly be saved, or helped, thanks to research with discarded embryos is not all that controversial. However, the first claim—that discarded embryos are going to die soon in any case—is far more controversial and has been challenged. I will thus focus on that claim in the next section.

Two versions of the nothing-is-lost principle

Will embryos discarded following IVF die soon in any case? According to Dan Brock the answer depends on how one understands 'in any case'.[24] Brock distinguishes a stronger and a weaker version of NILp. According to Brock, the stronger version 'implies that it could be permissible to kill a person who will die very soon anyway no matter what anyone does'.[25] Thus, the stronger version appeals to the fact that the loss

---

[23] Outka, 'Ethics of Embryonic Stem Cell Research', 595.
[24] Dan W. Brock, 'Creating Embryos for Use in Stem Cell Research', *Journal of Law and Medical Ethics*, 38 (2010), 229–37.
[25] Brock, 'Creating Embryos for Use', 232.

is going to occur *given what anyone could do*. In other words, *whatever anyone does*, the loss is going to occur. Brock rightly points out that the stronger version of NILp does not apply to discarded embryos as these embryos are frozen but still alive. Instead of being used for research, these embryos could remain frozen, or be given out for adoption and carried to term. It is thus not the case that these embryos are going to die given what anyone could do. Note that the stronger version of NILp does not apply to *Tim and the Indians* either. It is not the case that Mika is going to die given what anyone could do. The captain could, after all, modify his plan and instruct the soldiers not to kill any Indians.

The weaker version of NILp, as formulated by Brock, looks at 'what will happen given what others will *in fact* do' (implicitly assuming that the agent in question does nothing). Suppose that a researcher has been offered a frozen discarded embryo and is deliberating about whether to perform destructive research on it. Even though it is true that this embryo *could* be used for reproductive purposes if the researcher does nothing (that is, does not perform the research), it will not *in fact* be used for such purposes. If not used for research, it will instead be thawed and left to perish by the IVF clinic. It could be argued, then, that if the discarded embryo will not *in fact* be kept alive, nothing is lost by destroying it in research. Brock concludes that, although the weaker version of NILp *does* apply to the destruction of discarded embryos, it should not be accepted by those who accord a significant moral status to the embryo: accepting the destruction of a discarded embryo on this basis would be like accepting that a researcher who stumbles across an abandoned baby may use this baby in lethal medical research on the basis that it would have died anyway given what others will do. Brock rightly argues that the correct response in this situation is to care for the baby. He further concludes that

> those who rightly reject this weaker version of the nothing is lost principle will argue that likewise, the alternative to destroying spare embryos in hESC [human embryonic stem cell] research is to keep them alive and frozen or to give them to others for implantation.[26]

The weaker version of NILp, as formulated by Brock, is problematic indeed. The reason is that it looks at what others will do while assuming

---

[26] Brock, 'Creating Embryos for Use', 232.

that the person whose particular action is under moral consideration (henceforth 'the agent') *does nothing*, that is, (implicitly) assuming that she 'merely' abstains from causing the loss (for example, assuming that she merely abstains from killing the abandoned baby or the discarded embryo). But why does Brock understand the weaker version of NILp in a way that focuses only on *others*? In the stronger version of NILp, Brock includes *everyone's* future actions. The question there was whether the embryo could be saved by *anyone*, whether by the agent or by someone else. But Brock's formulation of the weaker version of NILp ignores positive steps the agent could take to prevent the loss and focuses only on others. I believe that any plausible version of NILp should *also* take into account the array of future actions open to the agent. Surely, if the agent could prevent the loss, she should (as Brock points out). If she does not prevent the loss, she contributes to the fact that something will be lost that would otherwise not have been lost. But there may be a situation where, even though others *could* prevent the loss, they in fact will not, and the agent cannot prevent the loss, or it is reasonable to assume she cannot. This is the case in *Tim and the Indians*: the captain and his soldiers could prevent Mika's death, but they will not. On the other hand, Tim cannot prevent the loss (recall that Tim wonders whether he could get hold of a gun but realizes that attempting this would result in all the Indians and himself being killed).

The mixed version of the nothing-is-lost principle

A plausible version of the nothing-is-lost principle, which *could* perhaps justify destroying a discarded embryo is what I call the 'mixed version'. The mixed version combines the stronger and weaker versions: it looks at what others will *in fact* do and at what the agent *could* do.

> *The Mixed Version of the Nothing-is-Lost principle (mixed NILp).* It is presumptively permissible to intentionally cause a loss that it would normally be impermissible to intentionally cause if (1) the loss is going to occur given what others will in fact do and regardless of what the agent does (from among the reasonable options), and (2) something good is expected to come out of causing the loss.

I believe that what is crucial to any version of NILp is that the expected loss is a *given* relative to the agent: a fixed baseline from which it is determined that no further loss is going to occur if the agent performs the action under moral consideration. Different versions of NILp can then be understood as specifying different conditions for taking a loss as a given relative to the agent. For example, in the stronger version, the loss can be taken as a given if it will occur whatever anyone does. In the mixed version, the loss can be taken as a given if it will occur whatever the agent does, where the actual actions of others are themselves taken as a given.

Recall the case of the sick tropical tree in your garden. Suppose your neighbour has the formula for producing a treatment for the diseased tropical tree. However, you have had problems with your neighbour for many years and, as a result, she refuses to give you the formula. Since you cannot find it elsewhere, you try to convince her to give it to you (by offering money, apologizing for past quarrels, etc.). However, you fail to change her mind. It seems somewhat plausible that, in this modified scenario, felling the tree could be justified by mixed NILp. The tree is going to die given what others will *in fact* do (refusing to share the formula), and regardless of what you do, from among the reasonable options, even though *someone*—your neighbour—could save it.

Applied to embryonic stem cell research, mixed NILp implies that it is presumptively permissible for a researcher to destroy an embryo if (1) the embryo is going to die soon given what others will in fact do and regardless of what the researcher[27] does (from among the reasonable options), and (2) something good is expected to come out of destroying the embryo.

The stronger version of NILp cannot justify destroying a discarded embryo, as it is not true that the embryo is going to die soon given what *anyone* could do. But could mixed NILp justify destroying a discarded embryo? Will a discarded embryo die given what others will in fact do and regardless of what the researcher does, from among the reasonable options? (Note that what options are reasonable will partly depend on what moral status one accords to the embryo.)

That a discarded embryo is going to die soon given what others will *in fact* do and assuming that the researcher in question does nothing is rather uncontroversial. The embryo has been donated for research because it was no longer wanted for reproductive purposes. If the

---

[27] I am assuming here that the agent is the researcher, as the question we are concerned with is whether it is permissible for a researcher to destroy an embryo to obtain stem cells (and not e.g. whether it is permissible for the state to finance embryonic stem cell research).

researcher does not use it, it will be thawed and left to perish by the IVF clinic, or it will be used by another researcher.

But will the embryo die regardless of what the researcher does? Not obviously. For example, as Brock has pointed out, the researcher may have the option of keeping the embryo alive and frozen or of donating the embryo to a couple who will use it for reproductive purposes.[28] It might indeed be thought that taking one or the other of these courses of action would prevent the loss from occurring. The first option—keeping the embryo frozen—is easier than the latter, but does it prevent the relevant loss?

What is the loss?

Whether the loss is going to occur in any case not only depends on the meaning of 'in any case'—the focus of Brock's analysis—but also on what exactly the relevant loss is that is going to occur in any case. So far, I have assumed that it is the life of a being of significant moral status: that of the particular embryo the researcher considers using for research. If this is indeed the loss, then keeping the embryo frozen prevents it, as the embryo remains alive.

However, perhaps the relevant loss is not the loss of the life of a being of significant moral status, but the loss of a *valuable* life of a being of significant moral status.[29] If that is indeed the loss then one does not necessarily prevent it by keeping the embryo in a freezer: one does not thereby enable the embryo to realize a life of value. Indeed, it might plausibly be thought that the loss of a valuable life is the *only* morally significant loss at stake here. The loss of life per se is not morally significant. In that case, retaining an embryo in a freezer (rather than destroying it in research) achieves nothing of moral importance.

Thus, it may be that, to prevent the loss, the researcher must do more than merely preserve the embryo in a freezer. Plausibly, she must ensure that the embryo is used for reproductive purposes, for example, by giving it to others for implantation. Is it *reasonable* to expect a researcher to do

---

[28] Brock, 'Creating Embryos for Use', 232.

[29] e.g. Don Marquis has famously argued that what makes killing wrong is that it deprives someone of a future of value. This applies to embryos too, regardless of their moral status. Don Marquis, 'Why Abortion is Immoral', *Journal of Philosophy*, 86 (1989), 183–202, and 'A Defence of the Potential Future of Value Theory', *Journal of Medical Ethics*, 28 (2002), 198–201.

this? Defenders of the discarded–created distinction must deny this. They typically refer to the current regulations and realities of IVF practices in most countries.[30] In the US alone about 600,000 embryos created in the context of fertility treatments are stored in nitrogen freezers. Many of these embryos, if no longer needed for reproductive purposes, will be donated to scientific research. Once an embryo has been donated to research, it would be illegal for the researcher to try to rescue it by giving it to an infertile couple. This is because the conceivers of the embryo only gave their consent for research use of their embryo, and not for reproductive use. The fact that it would be illegal for the researcher to rescue the embryo in this way suggests that it might not be a reasonable option for her to do so. Perhaps one could object that, even though it would be illegal to rescue the embryo in this way, the researcher is nevertheless *morally* required to give the embryo to a couple who is prepared to adopt it. The idea is that we should sometimes breach the law if that is required to save the life of a person. But even if this is so, it may be difficult for a researcher to find potential parents for the embryo, or a woman who is prepared to carry the embryo to term to then adopt it out. In the US, the National Embryo Donation Center and the Snowflakes Embryo Adoption Program have, with the consent of the conceivers of the embryos, arranged adoptions for some of the 600,000 frozen embryos. More than 400 children have been born through their programmes, but despite their best efforts to rescue frozen embryos, the great majority are not adopted. It could be argued then that if these organizations can hardly rescue any embryos, it is not a reasonable option for a researcher to do so. One could argue, of course, that if the researcher is a woman, she should rescue the embryo herself by carrying it to term. She could then either raise the child herself, or adopt it out once born. However, this implies that women are under a moral duty to carry embryos *in vitro* to term if they can, which is extremely controversial.[31]

---

[30] Outka, 'Ethics of Embryonic Stem Cell Research'. Ronald M. Green, 'Benefiting from "Evil": An Incipient Moral Problem in Human Stem Cell Research', *Bioethics*, 16 (2002), 544–56.

[31] Judith Jarvis Thomson—using the now famous violin thought experiment—has quite convincingly shown that even if a foetus (and thus an embryo) has a right to life, this does not imply it has a right to 'use' a woman's body to develop to term. Judith Jarvis Thomson, 'A Defense of Abortion', *Philosophy and Public Affairs*, 1 (1977), 47–66. According to Louis Guenin, women do not have 'a duty of intrauterine transfer'. This is because, according to Guenin, the burden of compelled parenthood or of compelled remote parenthood (in case

All this suggests that it is somewhat plausible to assume that it is not a reasonable option for a researcher to ensure that the embryo she considers using for research will be used for reproductive purposes instead. If the researcher cannot reasonably ensure the embryo is used for reproductive purposes, then it seems that mixed NILp *could* justify destroying a discarded embryo: it is going to die soon given what others will do and regardless of what the researcher does among the reasonable options. NILp would then imply that research on discarded embryos is presumptively permissible.

However, if this is true then mixed NILp could, at first sight, also justify the destruction of a *research* embryo. If a researcher who considers using a research embryo suddenly decided against doing so, the embryo would most likely be used by another researcher or it would be left to perish. It would die given what others will do (assuming the researcher does nothing). Moreover, it would die regardless of what the researcher does from among the reasonable options. After all, if it is true that a researcher cannot reasonably ensure a *discarded* embryo is used for reproductive purposes, then, for the same reasons, it must not be a reasonable option for a researcher to ensure a *research* embryo is used for reproductive purposes.[32]

So far, I have established that, contrary to what Brock has argued, it is not yet entirely ruled out that a plausible version of NILp—the mixed version—could justify deriving stem cells from discarded embryos if they are persons. However, I have also pointed out that, if that is true, it is also not yet ruled out that mixed NILp could justify deriving stem cells from research embryos. So how, then, could we back up the claim that NILp can presumptively justify destroying discarded embryos but not research embryos? What makes the crucial difference?

Nothing-is-lost and the destruction of research embryos

Some say that NILp cannot justify the destruction of research embryos 'since these embryos *need* not have been created for research in the

---

the new-born baby is adopted out) cannot be said to be reasonable when measured against the loss of the embryo's future life. Louis M. Guenin, *The Morality of Embryo Use* (Cambridge: Cambridge University Press, 2008), 189–90.

[32] Note that, as mentioned earlier, research embryos created through SCNT do not (yet) have this potential, which implies that even the stronger version of NILp could possibly apply to the destruction of these embryos. Since SCNT embryos may not be able to give rise to full-grown human beings in the near future, they are going to die soon, regardless of what anyone does.

first place'.[33] But this cannot be the whole story. After all, one could simply reply that surplus IVF embryos that are going to die in any case should not have been created in the first place either. If the embryo has a significant moral status, then how can it be justified to create many more embryos than will be needed to create a child via IVF, knowing that most of these embryos will be destroyed eventually? This needs to be justified too (I will return to this later). Moreover, once research embryos have been created, for example by researchers in a country with permissive stem cell policies, the question *remains* whether it is permissible for a researcher to make use of these embryos, or the products thereof. Thus, merely saying that research embryos should not have been created in the first place is not a satisfactory option for the defender of the discarded–created distinction.

Outka's specifications of the nothing-is-lost principle

Gene Outka gives a slightly fuller explanation for why he thinks NILp can justify destroying discarded embryos but not research embryos. According to Outka this

accords with the timbre of nothing is lost in that [in the case of discarded embryos] we encounter circumstances we did not initiate and that we wish were otherwise. That we contemplate doing repellent things that we would not do for their own sake indicates that intentional destroying was not 'part of our plan' from the start.[34]

As I specified NILp earlier, it holds that it is presumptively permissible for an agent to intentionally cause a loss that it is normally impermissible to intentionally cause if (i) the loss is going to occur in any case, and (ii) something good is expected to come out of causing the loss. The quoted passage from Outka could be read as introducing further conditions: that the agent (iii) should not have initiated the circumstances she encounters, (iv) should wish these circumstances were otherwise, and (v) did not plan to cause the loss 'from the start'.

Note that it is not clear how Outka's conditions relate to one another. Is it enough that one of these conditions obtains, or do they all need to obtain? Are they really separate conditions? It could be, for example, that

---

[33] See e.g. Brock, 'Creating Embryos for Use', 232.
[34] Outka, 'Ethics of Embryonic Stem Cell Research', 596.

what really matters to Outka is that it was not the researcher's plan to cause the loss all along, as specified by condition (v). Conditions (iii) and (iv) may be relevant only insofar as their satisfaction is evidence that condition (v) is also satisfied.

Rather than seeking to determine precisely which of these three conditions Outka would want to incorporate into his version of NILp, I will explore, in what follows, whether any of these conditions might allow him to offer a plausible variant of NILp that can justify destroying a discarded embryo but not a research embryo.

ONE SHOULD NOT HAVE INITIATED THE CIRCUMSTANCES ONE ENCOUNTERS

Presumably, Outka's idea in suggesting this condition is that a stem cell researcher who considers using a discarded embryo to obtain stem cells did not bring about the creation and discarding of that embryo. The embryo was created and discarded for reasons other than embryonic stem cell research. It was created in the context of a fertility treatment and discarded because no longer wanted for reproductive purposes. It is only given these circumstances, which the researcher did not initiate, that she considers using the embryo to obtain stem cells. It must then be assumed that a researcher who considers using a research embryo *did* initiate the creating and discarding of that embryo.

The question arises, however, why it matters, morally, whether one initiated the circumstances one encounters. Suppose that in *Tim and the Indians*, it was in fact Tim who captured and handed over the Indians to the captain, being perfectly aware of the fact that the latter would make him the wicked offer. When the captain makes the offer, Tim suddenly deeply regrets what he did. He does everything he can to reverse the circumstances, but alas, he cannot change the captain's plan. It seems possible that Tim's killing of Mika could still be justified under these circumstances, even though it was Tim who initiated them (and it was wrong to do so).

Likewise, it is plausible that mixed NILp could justify the destruction of a research embryo, even if the researcher initiated the circumstances she encounters (for example, by creating the embryo in circumstances which ensure its early death), but now regrets this and tries, without success, to prevent the loss.

ONE SHOULD WISH THE CIRCUMSTANCES
ONE ENCOUNTERS WERE OTHERWISE

Outka appears to be assuming here that a researcher using a discarded embryo wishes that the embryo was not going to die in any case. Indeed, according to Outka, the case for applying NILp to discarded embryos occurs in circumstances that are 'lamentable'. 'We welcome neither infertility nor excess embryos', he writes.[35] It must then be assumed that a researcher intending to use a research embryo does not think the circumstances are lamentable. Presumably the evidence for this is that she initiated the circumstances, and it was her plan to destroy the embryo all along.

But why exactly does it matter that the researcher wishes the circumstances she encounters were otherwise? Again, consider a modified version of Tim and the Indians where Tim in fact does not mind shooting Mika. Indeed it gives him a pleasurable feeling. Though it might be hypocritical of Tim to appeal to mixed NILp to justify shooting Mika[36] (as he does not consider Mika's death a loss and, perhaps does not think it would normally be impermissible to kill Mika), it is not immediately clear that from an objective viewpoint Tim's killing of Mika cannot be justified by mixed NILp. Likewise, it may not matter, from an objective viewpoint, whether or not the researcher regrets that the embryo she considers using is going to die in any case. Compare: it might be hypocritical for someone who believes that there is no right to freedom of religion to appeal to such a right in defending her religious practices. But it does not follow that there *is* no such right, nor that the person's practices could not be justified by that right.

CAUSING THE LOSS SHOULD NOT HAVE BEEN
THE PLAN ALL ALONG

The thought here seems to be that a researcher using a discarded embryo did not plan to destroy that embryo 'from the start', that is, presumably, from the moment the decision was made to create it. The embryo was created for reasons other than embryo research. By contrast, a researcher using a research embryo must have planned destroying the embryo from

---

[35] Outka, 'Ethics of Embryonic Stem Cell Research', 600.
[36] In his Tanner Lectures 'Incentives, Inequality and Community', Jerry Cohen (1991) argued that an argument's persuasive value may depend on who appeals to the argument. G. A. Cohen, 'Incentives, Inequality and Community', Stanford University, May 1991.

the start as the entire purpose of its creation was to use it in destructive research.

In *Tim and the Indians*, it clearly was not Tim's plan, prior to stumbling into the village, to kill Mika. But suppose it was his plan. Suppose he had come to the village with the intention of killing Mika. Why exactly would it be the case that NILp could no longer justify Tim's action? (Note that for it to have been Tim's plan all along to kill Mika, Tim need not have initiated or contributed to the circumstances he encounters. It might just be the case that the circumstances that obtain happen to be favourable to Tim realizing his plan to kill Mika.)

Again, it might be hypocritical of Tim to appeal to mixed NILp to justify shooting Mika. The fact that Tim planned killing Mika all along suggests he thinks killing an innocent person is permissible. But NILp is formulated as an exception to the rule that killing innocent persons is always wrong. It seems hypocritical, then, of Tim to appeal to NILp; this relies on a principle—killing innocent people is impermissible—that Tim is willing to disregard himself. However, it is not immediately clear that from an objective viewpoint Tim's killing of Mika cannot be justified by mixed NILp in this modified scenario.

Moreover, returning to embryonic stem cell research, it is not clear why a researcher using a research embryo must always have planned the destruction of that embryo from the start. True, if the researcher created the embryo herself, or requested its creation, this is quite strong evidence for the fact that she planned to destroy it all along. However, as has been pointed out, not every researcher using a research embryo must have created or requested its creation. A researcher could simply use a research embryo independently created by another researcher who no longer wishes to use it himself.

So, where does this leave us? Outka's criteria do not clearly license the conclusion that NILp cannot, from an objective viewpoint, justify any research on research embryos. Perhaps it might be possible to argue that some combination of Outka's conditions might work, but I think there is a more promising route to take.

The agency cost

So far I have ignored a potential problem that afflicts my formulation of NILp, as well as other standard formulations that appear in the literature. Suppose that in *Tim and the Indians*, the good that comes out of Tim shooting Mika is not that nineteen Indians are saved (there are no other Indians in this scenario), but that someone in a nearby village receives a free meal at the local restaurant (so the offer is: if Tim shoots Mika someone will get a free meal, if he does not shoot Mika, the soldiers will shoot Mika and no one will get a free meal). Intuitively it is much less clear that NILp could presumptively justify Tim's shooting of Mika in this modified scenario. Why is that? I suggest that, to explain this, we need to modify NILp by adding a condition. This condition holds that for NILp to justify an agent intentionally causing a loss that it would normally be impermissible to intentionally cause, the good that comes out of causing this loss must be proportionate to what I call the 'agency cost'. This is the moral cost of an agent being related in a certain way to the loss she causes, for example, the moral cost of the agent causing the loss, rather than merely allowing the loss to occur. Many (in particular those appealing to NILp) would think that there is a morally relevant difference between Tim shooting Mika, and Tim allowing the captain to shoot Mika; when Tim shoots Mika, his conduct possesses a wrong-making feature that it would not have possessed had he merely allowed the captain to shoot Mika. This might be understood as an instance of a more general moral difference between doing or causing and allowing harm. But the agency cost does not *need* to be understood in terms of the moral distinction between doing or causing and allowing; it might also be understood in terms of, for example, the moral distinction between direct versus indirect harmdoing, or intended versus merely foreseen harm; indeed, it may even be understood in terms of the adverse effects of the action on the agent's character.[37] For example, Michael Meyer and Lawrence Nelson write that

Whenever the forces of moral deliberation are called into play on behalf of an entity having even weak moral status, reasonable and conscientious persons clearly are required to give due regard to the entity in question *as well as to the manner in which their actions regarding it affect their own moral character* [emphasis added].

There is an agency cost whenever the agent's particular relationship to the loss that she causes constitutes a wrong-making feature of her

---

[37] Michael J. Meyer and Lawrence J. Nelson, 'Respecting What we Destroy: Reflections on Human Embryo Research', *Hastings Center Report*, 31 (2001), 18.

conduct, and the size of the cost is determined by the moral weight of this factor. It is this cost, I believe, which has to be proportionate to the good that comes out of the agent causing the loss. That is, I think, why it is implausible that NILp could justify Tim's destroying of Mika if the only good that came out of that was that someone in a nearby village receives a free meal. The good is not proportionate to the agency cost. It is not proportionate to the moral cost involved in the fact that Tim shoots Mika, instead of allowing the captain to shoot Mika.

If this is correct, then NILp should be modified as follows:

> *The Nothing-is-Lost principle (NILp).* It is presumptively permissible to intentionally cause a certain loss that it would normally be impermissible to intentionally cause if (1) the loss is going to occur in any case, (2) something good is expected to come out of causing the loss, and (3) the good that is expected to come out of causing the loss is proportionate to the agency cost.

So how could this help us find a justification for the view that NILp can justify destroying discarded embryos but not research embryos?

It may be the case that, when a researcher destroys a discarded embryo, condition (3) is met (the good that comes out of destroying the discarded embryo is proportionate to the agency cost), but that when a researcher destroys a research embryo condition (3) is not met.

Earlier, I pointed out that the good that is expected to come out of research with stem cells from research embryos is at least as great as the good that is expected to come out of research with stem cells from discarded embryos. Both types of embryonic stem cell research hold enormous promise for preventing or alleviating human suffering. Since the good that is expected to come out of destroying a research embryo and the good that is expected to come out of destroying a discarded embryo are equally large, it must be the agency cost that is different.

Though in both cases the researcher bears an agency cost because of her relationship to the present embryo's death—for example, in both cases the researcher destroys the embryo instead of allowing others to destroy it—there may be another wrong-making feature that is only present when a researcher destroys a research embryo, not when she destroys a discarded embryo. If this is so, the good that comes out of destroying a research embryo might be disproportionate to the agency cost involved in doing so, even though the same good would be proportionate to the agency cost involved in destroying a discarded embryo. The question is, then, what this additional wrong-making feature could be.

One important difference between *Tim and the Indians* and embryo research that I have ignored so far is that the latter is an ongoing practice rather than an individual action that is unlikely to be repeated. It is unlikely that the circumstances which Tim encounters will occur again, let alone recur on a regular basis. Thus, it is unlikely that Tim's response to the circumstances he encounters will have any effect on whether similar actions are performed in the future.

Embryonic stem cell research, however, is something that is typically done by researchers in a systematic way with legal endorsement. The circumstances in which (prospective) stem cell researchers find themselves are repeated over and over. This makes it much more likely that a single instance of destroying an embryo will have an effect on the future actions of others. It is this effect on others that I believe may help to explain why destroying a research embryo cannot be justified by NILp.

How does a researcher deriving stem cells from a research embryo influence the future actions of others, and how does this offer an explanation for why NILp cannot justify it?

The agency cost involved in destroying a research embryo

The most obvious way a researcher influences others' future actions by destroying a research embryo to obtain stem cells is by contributing to a demand for more research embryos, thereby encouraging the creation of embryos virtually doomed to never be used for reproductive purposes. To formulate it in Outka's terminology: even though the researcher did not contribute to 'the circumstances he encounters' now, by contributing to a demand for more research embryos he contributes to the existence of future circumstances similar to the ones he currently encounters: circumstances which virtually ensure that each research embryo is going to die given what others will do and regardless of what an individual researcher does. Through this mechanism, a researcher destroying a research embryo encourages further embryo deaths.

However, if the researcher abstained from destroying the embryo, and 'merely' allowed others to destroy it, surely further embryo deaths would also be encouraged, though not by the researcher in question. So whatever the researcher does, further embryo deaths will be encouraged. Why, then, can NILp not justify her destroying a research embryo? The reason is that the relationship between the researcher and the future losses she contributes to by destroying the embryo brings an agency cost to her action. The fact that she, rather than others, encourages further embryo deaths adds a wrong-making feature to her action, and this matters to those who appeal to NILp.

Thus, when a researcher destroys a research embryo, two losses occur—the loss of life of the present embryo and the loss of life of future embryos—and there is an agency cost associated with each. If the researcher does not destroy the embryo, both of these losses will still occur, but in neither case will the researcher bear any agency cost.

It could be argued, then, that when a researcher destroys a *research* embryo, the good that comes out of it is not proportionate to the agency cost, though it would be if the researcher were causing only a loss to the present embryo. If that is true, then the third condition of NILp is not met and NILp cannot justify deriving stem cells from research embryos. On the other hand, it might seem that NILp *can* justify the destruction of *discarded* embryos, since in this case there is no question of contributing to further embryo destruction. The discarded embryos are created, and doomed to death, by fertility doctors and their patients, and their actions are not influenced by the actions of researchers. As defenders of the discarded–created distinction have pointed out, discarded embryos exist and will continue to exist on a large scale regardless of whether embryonic stem cell research continues.[38] Ronald Green, for example, writes that

[t]he key insight here is that, at least at the present time and foreseeable future, embryo destruction is entirely independent of hESC research and therapy. Surplus embryos are routinely created in the practice of infertility medicine, where they result from current hyperstimulation regimes ... whatever some people choose to do, the massive creation and destruction of embryos will continue.[39]

[38] Green, 'Benefiting from Evil', 544–56. John A. Robertson, 'Causative vs. Beneficial Complicity in the Embryonic Stem Cell Debate', *Connecticut Law Review*, 36 (2003), 1099–113.
[39] Green, 'Benefiting from Evil', 554.

Green has compared the use and derivation of stem cells from discarded embryos to a variant of the oft appealed to 'murder victim case'.[40]

> *Murder Victim. A teen has been murdered in gang violence. After having obtained the consent of the teen's parents, a surgeon uses the murder victim's organs for transplantation into a patient who requires them in order to survive.*

Murder Victim is meant to draw out intuitions that will help us to determine when benefiting from others' wrongdoing is wrong itself. As I will discuss in more detail in the Chapter 3, it is generally thought that benefiting from others' wrongdoing may be wrong if this encourages similar wrongdoing in the future. Here we are indeed interested in whether destroying a discarded embryo, and thus benefiting from IVF practices, encourages further embryo destruction.

In Murder Victim we are meant to assume that benefiting from others' wrongdoing, in this case, a murder, will not encourage similar wrongdoing in the future. After all, it might seem extremely unlikely that the surgeon, by using the organs, will contribute to more gang murders. Thus, not only is nothing lost for the murder victim (or the brain-dead teen) by using his organs, no similar loss is caused to anyone else either. Moreover, someone will be saved. It seems that the surgeon's action could be justified by NILp. If using discarded embryos to obtain stem cells is similar to using organs from murder victims, then we should judge that it, too, can be justified by NILp.

But is using the organs from the brain-dead teen in Murder Victim analogous to the derivation of stem cells from discarded IVF embryos? If not, we cannot infer from the comparison that NILp can justify destroying discarded embryos. In the next section, I argue that deriving stem cells from discarded embryos is disanalogous to using the organs in Murder Victim and in such a way that it cannot be justified by NILp. I will base my analysis on Lynn Gillam's discussion of the analogy between Murder Victim and research on tissue obtained from aborted foetuses.

The agency cost involved in destroying a discarded embryo

In discussing whether the use of tissue from aborted foetuses is analogous to the use of organs from murder victims, Gillam distinguishes

---

[40] Green, 'Benefiting from Evil'. In Green's variant the victim has suffered brain death in the hospital after being grievously wounded in a 'drive by' gang shooting.

three mechanisms by which using the murder victim's organs might result in more murders: (1) by changing society's moral beliefs about murder, (2) by decreasing the state's efforts to deter it, and (3) by strengthening incentives to commit murder.[41] Gillam suggests that, because condemnation of murder is so deep-rooted in our moral psyche and is strongly reinforced by law worldwide, it is very unlikely that any of these effects will occur if we use organs from murder victims; it is therefore ethically permissible to do this. However, the circumstances of abortion differ from those of criminal murder: condemnation of abortion is not deeply rooted in almost everyone's intuitions, abortion legislation differs from country to country and has changed over time, and abortion is generally performed by the medical profession within a regulatory framework. These circumstances make it, according to Gillam, more likely that lobbying from pro-choice groups and the potential benefits of foetal tissue research will provide an incentive to relax existing abortion regulation or will result in reduced efforts to prevent abortion. In such a climate it may also be easier for women to justify their decision to abort their foetus. Gillam's point is that the differences in circumstances between abortion and criminal murder make it more likely that foetal tissue research will result in an increase in the number of abortions performed than that transplantation from murder victims will increase the murder rate. (Whether foetal tissue research actually *does* increase the abortion rate is extremely hard to establish as it is only one of several factors that may affect the abortion rate.)

Gillam points out that the circumstances of foetal tissue research and the murder victim case differ in a morally relevant way. I believe that Gillam's reasoning also applies to embryonic stem cell research as the circumstances are similar to those of foetal tissue research.[42] Defenders of the discarded-created distinction may be right that destroying discarded embryos does not directly create a demand for such embryos. However, as Gillam's analysis suggests, there are *other* mechanisms through which one may promote the destruction of embryos, for

---

[41] Lynn Gillam, 'Arguing by Analogy in the Fetal Tissue Debate', *Bioethics*, 11 (1997), 397–412.

[42] See also Tuija Takala and Matti Häyry, 'Benefiting from Past Wrongdoing, Human Embryonic Stem Cell Lines, and the Fragility of the German Legal Position', *Bioethics*, 21 (2007), 150–9.

example, by altering our attitudes to it or by taking away incentives to change certain practices so as to prevent the loss from reoccurring.

First, although a society that accepts IVF is unlikely to suddenly stop offering IVF treatments, it might still change the practice in such a way that fewer surplus embryos are created, and thus fewer embryos will be discarded. As I will explain in more detail, there are alternative ways to offer IVF, which do not involve the creation of surplus embryos for cryopreservation purposes. The benefits that flow from research using discarded embryos may weaken any incentive to implement or further develop such forms of IVF. Second, a researcher destroying a discarded embryo may also cause those already uncertain about the moral status of the embryo to feel increasingly comfortable about destroying embryos, making it easier to accept that embryos will not be used for reproduction, and reducing efforts to help 'rescue' embryos through embryo adoption. Finally, because embryonic stem cell research has the potential to benefit many more people than foetal tissue research, and the moral status of early embryos is generally less controversial than that of older foetuses, restrictions on the use of embryos for research and therapy (including fertility treatments) might be more easily loosened than the abortion regulations that Gillam has in mind.

Thus, it seems that, by destroying a discarded embryo, a researcher also contributes to the existence of future circumstances that are similar to the 'deplorable' circumstances she currently encounters. As a result, a researcher destroying a discarded embryo also contributes to further embryo deaths. This adds the same wrong-making feature to the researcher's action as in the case of a researcher destroying a research embryo. Both types of research seem to involve the same agency cost, for they both involve (i) intentionally causing the present embryo to die, and (ii) foreseeably contributing to future embryo deaths.

Unless there is another reason why the agency cost of a researcher destroying a research embryo is significantly higher than the agency cost of a researcher destroying a discarded embryo (and it is now up to the defender of the discarded–created distinction to show this), we should accept that if the good that comes out of destroying a research embryo is not proportionate to the agency cost, then the good that comes out of destroying a discarded embryo must not be proportionate to the agency cost either. Thus, if NILp fails to justify destroying research embryos because the proportionality condition is not satisfied, it also fails to justify destroying discarded embryos, for the same reason.[43] If, on the other hand, one believes the good that comes out of destroying a discarded embryo *is* proportionate to the agency cost, then one must accept that the same is true for destroying a research embryo. Either way, NILp cannot support the discarded−created distinction. The principle either presumptively justifies both research on discarded embryos and research on research embryos, or it justifies neither.

But perhaps I am being too quick here. One could object to my analysis that there is indeed something else that significantly increases the agency cost involved when a researcher destroys a research embryo. This could be so if it is significantly worse to encourage the creation of embryos virtually doomed to die in the context of embryonic stem cell research than it is to encourage the creation of embryos doomed to die in the context of IVF. What needs to be shown then is that it is significantly worse to create research embryos than it is to create surplus IVF embryos that are likely to be discarded. If this is so then it could be argued that the agency cost involved in destroying a research embryo might not be outweighed by the good that is expected to come out of it, even though the agency cost associated with destroying a discarded embryo *can* be outweighed by the good that is expected to come out of it. In this way one might be able to rescue the nothing-is-lost argument.

In what follows, I discuss two arguments that have been adduced to show that the creation and destruction of embryos for research is worse than the creation and destruction of embryos in the context of IVF. One argument appeals to the Doctrine of Double Effect, and another to the respect we owe to the embryo. Note that even though these arguments, if they succeed, could rescue the nothing-is-lost argument, they have been

---

[43] I have been assuming that the good that is expected to come out of research using a research embryo and the good that is expected to come out of research using a discarded embryo are equally large. However, given that research with research embryos could solve problems that research with discarded embryos cannot solve, the good that is expected to come out of that research could be said to be larger than the good expected to come out of research with discarded embryos. This suggests that, even if the agency cost would be somewhat greater when a researcher destroys a research embryo than when she destroys a discarded embryo, this cost might still be outweighed by the larger expected benefits of the research. Thus, defenders of the discarded−created distinction would have to show that the agency cost associated with a researcher destroying a research embryo is significantly higher than that associated with a researcher destroying a discarded embryo; a task, I believe, in which they have not succeeded thus far. I return to this issue in Chapter 5.

adduced as separate arguments in defence of the discarded–created distinction. If they do not work as separate arguments, as I hope to show, then, obviously, they cannot rescue the nothing-is-lost argument either. After all, if they fail to show that the creation and destruction of research embryos is significantly worse than the creation and destruction of discarded embryos then we have reason to believe that the agency cost involved when a researcher destroys a research embryo is the same as, or very similar to, the agency cost involved when a researcher destroys a discarded embryo.

2.5. Double Effect

The survival lottery

What defenders of the discarded–created distinction find of crucial importance is that, unlike research embryos, discarded embryos were created with the intention to have a child. This is sometimes used to support the view that embryo loss in IVF is like embryo loss in 'natural' or sexual reproduction. The majority of embryos created in sexual reproduction die spontaneously within a few weeks of conception, with the riskiest time being that before implantation into the uterine wall. According to some estimates, a mother of three children could be expected to have also had approximately five spontaneous abortions.[44] As John Harris famously framed it, 'sexual reproduction is a survival lottery'.[45] Some have argued that IVF is a similar kind of survival lottery.

For example, several members of the President's Council on Bioethics wrote that

[p]recisely because one cannot tell which IVF embryo is going to reach the blastocyst stage, implant itself in the uterine wall, and develop into a child, the embryo 'wastage' in IVF is more analogous to the embryo wastage in natural sexual intercourse practice by a couple trying to get pregnant than it is to the creation and use of embryos that requires (without exception) their destruction.[46]

---

[44] Toby Ord, 'The Scourge: Moral Implications of Natural Embryo Loss', *American Journal of Bioethics*, 7 (2008), 12–19.

[45] John Harris, 'Sexual Reproduction is a Survival Lottery', *Cambridge Quarterly of Healthcare Ethics*, 13 (2004), 75–89.

[46] President's Council on Bioethics, *Human Cloning and Human Dignity: An Ethical Inquiry* (Washington, DC: President's Council on Bioethics, 2002), ch. 6, s. 4.

The conclusion that has been drawn then is that, if embryo loss in IVF is similar to that in sexual reproduction, it must be permissible, even if the embryo is a person. After all, even those who accord a full moral status to the embryo think sexual reproduction is permissible.

However, some have argued that it is inconsistent to at the same time believe that the embryo is a person *and* to accept natural reproduction, given that it involves such a large embryo loss.[47] The idea is that if one really believes the embryo is a person, one should not create and 'sacrifice' embryos in order to have a child.

One argument that has been advanced to show that sexual reproduction is nevertheless permissible if embryos are persons appeals to the Doctrine of Double Effect. Thomas Aquinas is credited with introducing Double Effect in his discussion of the permissibility of self-defence. Suppose an agent wants to protect her own life and can only do so by killing her assailant. Although Aquinas believed that there is an absolute moral prohibition against killing persons, he argued that killing the assailant may nevertheless be permissible if the *intention* is self-defence and if the act of killing is in proportion to the end. Killing the assailant would be impermissible, for example, if more violence is used than is required to defend oneself.[48]

Double Effect has evolved into a principle that can be invoked to provide moral guidance in a situation where an agent wishes to do good, but cannot do so without causing serious harm. It holds that it may be permissible to bring about a harm as a foreseen but unintended side-effect of an action that is aimed at some good end (for example, the creation of a child), even though it is impermissible to bring about the same harm as a *means* to achieve that end.

Disagreement about the meaning and function of Double Effect has resulted in various formulations of the doctrine, but they all have in common the idea that the permissibility of bringing about certain kinds

---

[47] Dan W. Brock, 'Is a Consensus Possible on Stem Cell Research? Moral and Political Obstacles', *Journal of Medical Ethics*, 32 (2006), 36–42. Harris, 'Sexual Reproduction is a Survival Lottery'. Robert Sparrow and David Cram, 'Saviour Embryos? Preimplantation Genetic Diagnosis as a Therapeutic Technology', *Reproductive BioMedicine Online*, 20 (2010), 667–74.

[48] Thomas Aquinas, *Summa Theologica* II-II, q. 64, art. 7, 'Of Killing', in Richard J. Regan and William P. Baumgarth (eds), *On Law, Morality, and Politics* (Indianapolis and Cambridge: Hackett Publishing Co, 1988), 226–7.

of harm hinges on a number of conditions being met. An influential version in medical ethics is that of Joseph Mangan. According to this version, for an action that has both a good and a bad effect to be permissible, four conditions need to be met:

(1) That the action in itself from its very object be good or at least indifferent;
(2) That the good effect and not the evil effect be intended;
(3) That the good effect be not produced by means of the evil effect;
(4) That there be a proportionately grave reason for permitting the evil effect.[49]

Timothy Murphy has argued that embryo loss in sexual reproduction can be justified by Double Effect.[50] Murphy focuses on the intention, the means, and the proportionality criteria of double effect. (He is silent on the first criterion. Since I can also make my point without reference to this criterion, I will be silent on it too.)

Murphy basically argues that sexual reproduction is permissible because (i) the intention is to create a child, and not to expose embryos to risk, (ii) embryo loss is not a means to creating a child as it is possible that a child is created without any embryos dying along the way and, moreover, the embryos do not die in order to ensure that other embryos will make it, and (iii) the good of bringing new life into the world is proportionate to the loss of life.

If embryo loss in IVF is like embryo loss in sexual reproduction, and embryo loss in sexual reproduction can be justified by Double Effect, then embryo loss in IVF should also be justifiable by an appeal to Double Effect. Indeed this is what Murphy and some defenders of the discarded–created distinction have argued.

Murphy writes that

[a]s a matter of double-effect reasoning, however, a prima facie case can be made in defence of conception in vitro for fertility medicine, since no objectionable motives are involved, the objectionable effect is not the means by which the desirable effect is achieved, and there is an important benefit from IVF that

[49] Joseph Mangan, 'An Historical Analysis of the Principle of Double Effect', *Theological Studies*, 10 (1949), 43.
[50] Timothy M. Murphy, 'Double-Effect Reasoning and the Conception of Human Embryos', *Journal of Medical Ethics*, doi:10.1136/medethics-2012-100534.

counterbalances any undesirable outcome. The same cannot be said of conception in vitro for the purposes of any research that destroys embryos... [51]

Dan Brock also argues that Double Effect could plausibly be appealed to
by defenders of the discarded–created distinction (though Brock himself
does not accept Double Effect):

Defenders of the doctrine of double effect might argue that all [IVF embryos] are
created for the purpose of reproduction, but with a possible foreseen consequence that not all will be needed for that purpose; the creation of excess embryos
that might be used in research is foreseen as a possible consequence, but is not
intended. [52]

Brock further writes that

On the other hand, in using IVF with no reproductive intent and solely to create
embryos for use in research, their destruction is intended and not merely
foreseen.

In a similar vein, Jacques Suaudeau, from the Pontifical Academy for
Life, writes on research using research embryos that

[T]his shocking act does not come in association with the beneficial act, or as a
side effect not sought as such, but is the basic condition for the good effect
sought. This excludes application of the principle of double effect (indirectly
voluntary) to therapeutic cloning. [53]

If this is all true, then there is nothing morally problematic about the
creation of surplus IVF embryos that will likely be discarded. The
nothing-is-lost principle might then further justify the use of these
embryos for stem cell derivation purposes. Although the destruction of
discarded embryos encourages subsequent creation of surplus embryos
destined to be discarded, this is not a problem, as the creation of such
embryos is itself permissible. The discarded–created distinction would be
a valid ethical position. But can the creation of IVF embryos that are
likely to be discarded be justified by Double Effect? [54] I am myself

---

[51] Murphy, 'Double-Effect Reasoning', 3.

[52] Brock, 'Creating Embryos for Use', 233.

[53] J. Suaudeau, 'From Embryonic Stem Cells to iPS: An Ethical Perspective', *Cell Proliferation*, 44 (2011), 70–84.

[54] The section on Double Effect is partly based on Katrien Devolder, 'Embryo Deaths in Reproduction and Embryo Research: A Reply to Murphy's Double Effect Argument', *Journal of Medical Ethics* (2012) doi:10.1136/medethics-2012-101065.

sceptical of the normative force of Double Effect, but for the sake of argument I assume here that it is a valid principle.

Proportionality

A first problem with the argument is that it is implausible that the discarding, and thus the destruction, of discarded embryos is an *unintended side-effect* of IVF. That some embryos are surplus *may* be an unintended side-effect of IVF, but these embryos could be donated to infertile couples to be carried to term (or be kept frozen, though as I have already argued, on some views this may not prevent harming the embryo). That these embryos are instead donated for research is the result of further choices that intentionally lead to the embryos' destruction. (Also note that it must be clear now that the destruction of embryos to obtain stem cells—so not their 'mere' discarding—cannot be justified by Double Effect, as this involves an even further decision, a decision to intentionally use the embryo as a source of stem cells.)

But suppose, as we have before and as is somewhat plausible, that giving surplus embryos up for adoption is not an option (say, because there is not enough demand). Now, plausibly, the discarding and thus destruction of these embryos would be merely a foreseen but unintended side-effect of the parents' efforts to have a child. There is no further decision to discard them, rather than adopt them out. So if the discarding of surplus IVF embryos is an unintended side-effect, can Double Effect justify the creation of surplus IVF embryos that will likely be discarded? I believe it cannot.

For Double Effect to apply more is required than that the agents bring about the harm as an unintended side-effect of promoting a good end. On most standard versions, including the one invoked by Murphy, it requires that some kind of proportionality condition has been satisfied (condition 4 in Mangan's version). Indeed, Aquinas made the proportionality condition part of Double Effect when stating that killing the assailant in self-defence is impermissible if more violence is used than is required to defend oneself. Alan Donagan explains the proportionality condition as follows:

Whether or not the good effect is a proportionately serious reason is determined according to the principle that evil is to be avoided or prevented wherever possible, except at the cost of an equal or worse evil. If the nonoccurrence of the good effect would be as great an evil, or a worse evil, than the occurrence of the bad effect, then it is a proportionately serious reason for it.[55]

Murphy argues that in IVF, as in sexual reproduction, 'the unwanted loss of some embryonic life seems counterbalanced by the desirable generation of new lives'.[56] It is indeed plausible that the bad side-effect of unintended embryo deaths, whether in sexual reproduction or in IVF, is less bad than a situation in which no new children are brought into the world. To illustrate this, we can simply compare these deaths with the death of some of the children we bring into the world. Even though we know that typically some of our children may die prematurely, we accept this risk in order to have children. We generally think that the good of bringing children into the world outweighs the badness of some of them dying prematurely. However, applying the proportionality condition is not as straightforward as Murphy seems to think. His analysis may be correct if applied to certain IVF practices that do indeed resemble sexual reproduction (at least, if the proportionality condition is met in sexual reproduction—this is controversial). However, it clearly fails when applied to IVF as it is practised in most countries. If we apply it to standard IVF practices, then Murphy is comparing the wrong things. I will illustrate this with a hypothetical case in a different context. Consider

Road Building. The city council decides to build a road. To achieve this end, ten road workers will have to construct the road, three of whom are likely to die as a result of the hard labour (and we don't know beforehand who will die). The works will take a year to complete. The alternative is not building the road, in which case no one will die.

In this case, the good end is the completion of a new road in one year's time, and the harm that occurs as a result is the death of three workers. To see whether the proportionality condition is met, we have to ask whether the badness of the death of three workers is proportionate to the badness of not achieving the good end—the completion of a new road. What we are comparing then is the absolute benefit (a new road) with the absolute harm, that is, the death of three workers. (I am assuming it

[55] Alan Donagan, *The Theory of Morality* (Chicago: University of Chicago Press, 1977), 161.
[56] Murphy, 'Double-Effect Reasoning', 3.

would be worse if the road was not built at all.) Likewise we could, as Murphy does, compare doing IVF with not doing IVF at all. To see whether the proportionality condition is met, we would compare the absolute benefit (creating a child via IVF) with the absolute harm that occurs as a result (the death of a number of embryos). It seems to me, however, that we would then be comparing the wrong things.

I have already explained where discarded embryos that are used to obtain stem cells come from. In most countries where IVF is practised, on average five to ten embryos are produced per IVF cycle, one or two of which are transferred to the woman's uterus to try to achieve a pregnancy. The remaining embryos are stored in nitrogen freezers. If an attempt to achieve a pregnancy fails, one or two embryos can be thawed for a new attempt. Cryopreservation of several embryos has the advantage that women do not have to undergo the hormone therapy and egg retrieval procedure, which entail some risk and discomfort after each failed attempt to generate a pregnancy. Recall that at the start of the IVF treatment, the couple must indicate one of the following options for handling of any leftover frozen embryos: (1) donation to other infertile couples, (2) donation to scientific research, or (3) allowing the embryos to perish. The two last options both involve the embryo's destruction.

I will call this type of IVF *woman-friendly* IVF, because in this type of IVF, embryos are exposed to major risks for the benefit of the woman undergoing IVF. But IVF can also be done without the creation of surplus embryos likely to be consigned to death. Some countries allow IVF but prohibit the creation of extra embryos for cryopreservation purposes. For example, Italy limits the number of oocytes that can be fertilized to three and all embryos created *in vitro* have to be transferred to the woman's uterus. I will refer to IVF as it is done in Italy—without the creation of surplus embryos for cryopreservation purposes—as *embryo-friendly* IVF.[57]

So now that it is clear that the options include not merely woman-friendly IVF and no IVF, but also embryo-friendly IVF, let us return to

---

[57] A more recent development in IVF is to freeze eggs, instead of embryos, and to then thaw the eggs to fertilize them *in vitro* after each failed attempt to generate a pregnancy. This method is still experimental in Europe, but has been used in the clinic elsewhere. In Italy freezing eggs may become an alternative to implanting all the embryos created. This would reduce the risk of twin or triplet pregnancies significantly.

the proportionality principle of Double Effect. (Recall that, for the moment, we are assuming the embryo is a person, as Murphy does.)

Consider a variant of Road Building:

Road Building*. The city council decides to build a road. There are two options. The first option is as in Road Building. It involves building the road with ten workers, three of whom are likely to die. The works will take a year to complete. The second option is to build the road with ultramodern machines and only three road workers, none of whom will die. The works will take one year and four months to complete. All other things are equal.

If this alternative—building the road less quickly but without any deaths—is available, then it seems we should think of the good end and side-effects in a relative way. Now we should construe the good effect as building the road *four months more quickly* and the harmful side-effect as *three human deaths instead of none*. It seems clear that the city council should choose the second option. The cost of losing three human lives is, all other things being equal, just too high to justify the benefit of finishing the road works four months earlier. The relative benefit is too small to justify the relative harm.

If we take the same approach for woman-friendly IVF, we need to compare it with embryo-friendly IVF instead of with not doing IVF at all. The good effect of doing woman-friendly IVF will then not be the creation of a child (a child will be created either way), but the reduced health risks and discomfort for the woman undergoing IVF. So just like in *Road Building*, there is an alternative to achieving the good end that is less safe and convenient (in this case, for the woman undergoing IVF). The crucial question, then, is whether the relative benefit of woman-friendly IVF is large enough to outweigh the badness of the embryo deaths.[58]

What are the relevant benefits of woman-friendly IVF? It reduces the average number of IVF cycles the woman will have to undergo to have

---

[58] If we apply this analysis to sexual reproduction, the question is whether there is an alternative to current (embryo-unfriendly) natural reproduction (apart from not reproducing at all). One could argue that such an alternative is possible, if only we invested more time and effort in it. For example, if we did more research into causes and prevention of spontaneous abortion, we could make sexual reproduction more embryo-friendly. The difference with embryo-friendly IVF is that, at the moment, there is no embryo-friendly sexual reproduction. It would be interesting to investigate whether my argument also applies to sexual reproduction. However, this is beyond the scope of this book's aim.

a baby, thereby reducing the cost, and the physical and psychological burden for the woman and her partner. Woman-friendly IVF also obviates the need for the woman to take a hormone treatment to stimulate her ovaries to produce eggs, and to undergo the egg retrieval procedure after each failed attempt to achieve a pregnancy. The hormone treatment and egg retrieval procedure involve risks and inconveniences that are mostly mild but in some cases can be severe. One of the more serious possible effects of the hormone treatment is the development of the ovarian hyperstimulation syndrome (OHSS), which may involve abdominal swelling and pain, nausea, vomiting, and sometimes diarrhoea, and which may vary in severity. In rare cases it is lethal. Finally, probably the most important advantage of woman-friendly IVF over embryo-friendly IVF is that it reduces the risk of a twin or triplet pregnancy, which comes with an increased risk of harm for both the woman and the foetuses.

Although the risks and inconveniences should not be underestimated, surely, one would not normally impose life-threatening risks on persons to reduce this sort of risk and inconvenience.

Indeed we would not sacrifice those with a full moral status even if the risks were higher than those in IVF treatment. Consider the following hypothetical case:

> *Frozen Babies.* Sonya and Steve want a child. Making use of IVF they produce eight viable embryos, one of which is randomly chosen for transfer to Sonya's uterus. The remaining seven embryos, instead of being cryopreserved, are carried to term by surrogate mothers. After birth, the seven babies are (painlessly) frozen. The reason is that should something bad happen to Sonya's baby at birth or shortly afterwards, one of the frozen babies can be thawed and given to her. Sonya would thereby be spared from having to undergo the IVF procedure and the pregnancy again. Fortunately nothing goes wrong. Sonya and Steve do not want more than one baby, and decide to donate the frozen babies to scientific research that involves a process that will kill the babies.

Suppose that Sonya and Steve do not have the choice to adopt out the frozen babies (just like we have assumed it is not possible for a couple undergoing IVF to donate their frozen embryos to infertile couples). It is intuitively clear that Double Effect cannot justify discarding, and thus killing, the frozen babies, and I believe that the reason is that the proportionality condition is not met. Imposing such serious risks on the babies is out of proportion to the good effect of creating frozen babies—that is, potentially avoiding the need for Sonia to undergo another IVF procedure, pregnancy, and delivery if the first baby does not survive. If Double Effect cannot justify the special IVF procedure Sonya and Steve are using, then, by analogy, it cannot justify woman-friendly IVF either. If the proportionality condition is not met in *Frozen Babies*, then surely it is not met in woman-friendly IVF. After all, the risks imposed on the embryos are to prevent a smaller harm (risks from IVF) in woman-friendly IVF than in *Frozen Babies* (risks from IVF, pregnancy, and the delivery) and the costs are the same.

So far, we have been assuming an embryo has a full moral status. Of course, one could deny that the embryo has a full moral status and still believe that the embryo is worthy of moral consideration. If we assume that the embryo has a lower intermediate moral status, it is less clear whether the creation and discarding of embryos in the context of IVF is in proportion to the good that is produced through IVF. This will depend on how high one thinks the embryo's intermediate moral status is. If one thinks it is very high (for example, just a bit lower than that of a person), then the harm to the embryo should also be considered out of proportion to the good effect, that is, preventing or reducing harm to women undergoing IVF. On the other hand, if one thinks the embryo's moral status is low enough for the creation and destruction of discarded embryos to be proportionate to the good effect of reducing harm to women undergoing IVF, it becomes very difficult to explain why the creation and destruction of research embryos is impermissible given that it could significantly benefit a large number of people. The benefit of reducing health risks to a woman undergoing IVF seems smaller than the benefit of embryonic stem cell research with research embryos.

Once we assume that the embryo has a lower moral status, there is, however, another argument that could show that it is significantly worse to create and destroy embryos for research than to create and destroy embryos in the context of assisted reproduction. If this argument succeeds, then it could justify the discarded–created distinction, either as a separate argument, or as part of the nothing-is-lost argument (it would show that the agency cost involved in destroying a research embryo is significantly greater than the agency cost involved in destroying discarded embryo because it is significantly worse to encourage the creation and destruction of research embryos than to encourage the creation and destruction of discarded embryos).

2.6. Respect

The argument I have in mind holds that using discarded embryos to obtain stem cells is part of a practice—IVF—that treats the embryo, over the course of its whole life, with respect, whereas using research embryos to obtain stem cells is part of a practice that treats the embryo disrespectfully. The obvious question that arises is what is meant by respectful treatment in this context and how it could be the case that research embryos are not treated with respect, whereas embryos created in the context of IVF but subsequently destroyed in research are? Indeed, how is it that one can have respect for something that one intentionally destroys?

Respecting what we destroy

Recall the official Roman Catholic view that

> The human being is to be respected and treated as a person from the moment of conception; and therefore from that same moment his rights as a person must be recognized, among which in the first place is the inviolable right of every innocent human being to life.[59]

If respect for persons entails that one should recognize each person's right to life, as the Roman Catholic Church asserts, then destroying discarded embryos is incompatible with respectful treatment. It would violate the embryo's right to life. As already argued, the nothing-is-lost argument cannot convincingly justify killing discarded embryos if the embryo has a full moral status.

However, if the embryo has a lower intermediate moral status then it is much more plausible that we could treat it with respect even though we destroy it. Simply compare this with how we treat animals. Most people accord an intermediate moral status to animals. Still, many think that killing animals does not necessarily involve treating them with disrespect. Whether we treat animals with respect may depend on certain conditions, such as whether we only kill them for important purposes, whether there are alternative ways of achieving our goals without harming beings with an equally high, or a higher moral status, whether we

---

[59] Pope John Paul II's *Evangelium Vitae* encyclical (1995), with reference to the *Donum Vitae*, and updated in *Dignitas Personae* (2008 n. 4) instruction of the Congregation for the Doctrine of Faith (1987).

kill them as painlessly as possible, and so forth. Another example of respectful treatment that can go together with destruction is research with cadavers. Even though cadavers are sometimes destroyed in medical research, we can still treat them respectfully.[60] What respectful treatment of animals or cadavers entails is of course open for further discussion.

Now that we have established that if the embryo has an intermediate moral status, destroying it plausibly need not involve treating it with disrespect, the relevant question is why it is that the creation and destruction of discarded embryos, but not of research embryos, is compatible with respectful treatment. What makes the difference?

Unfortunately, the notion of respect is often invoked without much explanation or argumentation.[61] It is rarely explained why a certain kind of behaviour or certain attitudes amount to disrespectful treatment of the embryo. I will, however, attempt to reconstruct some of the statements that have been made into arguments that could, at first sight, support the discarded–created distinction.

Treating the embryo as an end, not merely as a means

Immanuel Kant famously argued that respecting a person entails treating that person as an end in itself and never merely as means.[62] This implies that we should never treat a person as if she had value only insofar as she is useful to us. Some seem to have this Kantian notion of respect in mind when defending the view that there is a moral difference between the way discarded and research embryos are treated.

For example, Axel Kahn writes that

the creation of human clones solely for spare cell lines would, from a philosophical point of view, be in obvious contradiction to the principle expressed by Emmanuel Kant: that of human dignity. This principle demands that an individual—and I would extend this to read human life—should never be thought of as a means, but always also as an end.[63]

---

[60] For more examples of things we at the same time respect and can permissibly destroy, see Meyer and Nelson, 'Respecting What we Destroy'.

[61] M. Therese Lysaught, 'Respect: Or, How Respect for Persons Became Respect for Autonomy', *Journal of Medicine and Philosophy*, 29 (2004), 665–80.

[62] Stephen L. Darwall, 'Two Kinds of Respect', *Ethics*, 88 (1977), 36–49.

[63] Axel Kahn, 'Clone Mammals . . . Clone Man?', *Nature*, 336 (1997) and 'Cloning, Dignity and Ethical Revisionism', *Nature*, 388 (1997), 320.

Several members of the US President's Council on Bioethics agreed that,

> [E]ven though [in IVF] more eggs are fertilized than will be transferred to a woman, each embryo is brought into being as an end in itself, not simply as a means to other ends.[64]

Similarly, William FitzPatrick writes that creating research embryos

> seems to involve a distinct kind of exploitative attitude, reflecting the thought that an embryo is something whose entire significance may be characterized by the external purposes for which we brought it into existence—the clearest possible case of treating something as a 'mere means'.[65]

However, as has been pointed out numerous times before,[66] the Kantian notion of respect 'that one should always treat someone as an end and not merely as a means' does not apply to early embryos, let alone to embryos that do not yet exist (most seem to object to '*bringing* embryos *into being*' simply as a means to other ends). Kant's principle instructs us to take seriously the rationality of persons by respecting them as ends. However, embryos, regardless of their moral status, lack rationality. Hence they cannot be the subject of Kantian respect.

Although the Kantian notion of respect does not strictly apply to embryos, the references to 'using something as an end and not merely as a means' may, of course, be indicative of other important considerations regarding respectful treatment. The question is of which ones. For example, what can someone mean when claiming that embryos in IVF are treated as an end?

The prospect of living

Consider this passage from the House of Lords 2002 report on stem cell research.[67]

---

[64] President's Council on Bioethics, *Human Cloning and Human Dignity*, ch. 6, s. 4.

[65] William FitzPatrick, 'Surplus Embryos, Nonreproductive Cloning, and the Intend/ Foresee Distinction', *Hastings Center Report*, 33 (2003), 30.

[66] See e.g. Dena S. Davis, 'Embryos Created for Research Purposes', *Kennedy Institute of Ethics Journal*, 5 (1995), 343–54. Bonnie Steinbock, 'What does "Respect for Embryos" Mean in the Context of Stem Cell Research?', *Women's Health Issues*, 10 (2000), 127–30.

[67] House of Lords, Select Committee on Stem Cell Research,. *Stem Cell Research: Report* (London: House of Lords, 2002), ch. 4, s. 4.27.

But most of those who commented on this issue regarded it as preferable to use surplus embryos than to create them specifically for research. They took the view that an embryo created for research was quite clearly being used as a means to an end, with no prospect of implantation, whereas at the time of creation the surplus embryo had a prospect of implantation, even if, once not selected for implantation (or freezing), it would have to be destroyed.

This passage suggests that many think that what determines that discarded embryos are treated with respect ('as an end and not merely as means') is the fact that each discarded embryo at the time of creation has 'a prospect of implantation' even if, once not selected for implantation, it will be discarded. Research embryos do not have this prospect. From the moment a research embryo comes into existence it is virtually determined that it will be destroyed in research. After all, that is why it was brought into existence in the first place.

But is it really the fact that an embryo has the prospect of further development which makes it the case that we treat it with respect? Consider the following scenario. Suppose each time we create a batch of research embryos we randomly select some for donation to infertile couples. At the time of their creation, each research embryo would, then, have the prospect of developing into a baby. This would be true even if we randomly selected only one embryo for use in a reproductive project. If we adopted such a scheme, would we then be treating research embryos with respect? If so, then the only thing we need to do to make the creation and use of research embryos permissible is change the practice according to this scheme.[68]

However, many who accord an intermediate moral status to the embryo (remember, we have already shown that the argument of respect cannot justify embryo destruction if the embryo is a person) would argue that this would fail to express respect for the embryo because, even though each of the embryos has a chance to develop into a child, they are really created because that is the best way to promote research. Treating an embryo with respect requires that it is created with the *intention* to have a child, as in sexual reproduction where the intention

---

[68] John Harris and Julian Savulescu have referred to similar lotteries. John Harris, 'Survival Lottery' in John Harris (ed.), *Bioethics* (New York: Oxford University Press, 2001), 300–15. Julian Savulescu, 'The Embryonic Stem Cell Lottery and the Cannibalization of Human Beings.', *Bioethics*, 16 (2002), 508–29.

is to have a child, but where some embryos may die in the course of pursuing that goal.

The intention to have a child

The intention with which embryos are created in the course of an IVF treatment is the creation of a child. At the time of the creation of the embryos, it is not known which, if any, of the embryos will become that child. By contrast, research embryos are not created with the intention to produce a child. Even if we organized a lottery like the one just suggested, the intention would not be to create a child, but to advance the field of stem cell research.

But how exactly does the fact that discarded embryos were created with the intention to bring a child into the world relate to respectful treatment? Consider again the earlier discussed Frozen Babies case. Though the intention of Sonya and Steve is to have a child, it seems intuitively clear that the frozen babies are not treated respectfully. There are two reasons for why this is so. First, Sonya and Steve decide to donate the frozen babies to research instead of giving them a chance to live (for example, by giving them up for adoption). I pointed out that perhaps Sonya and Steve do not have a choice because, say, there is not enough demand for adoption. But even then it seems intuitively clear that their actions are disrespectful. Imposing such grave risks on the babies (by creating many more than will likely be needed) is out of proportion to the good effect—preventing or reducing harm to Sonya due to the IVF procedure, the pregnancy, and the delivery. Since Frozen Babies is analogous to standard IVF practices, we can conclude that embryos, if they are persons, are not treated with respect in these practices either, even though they were created with the intention to bring a child into the world.

However, we are assuming now that the embryo has a lower intermediate moral status so Frozen Babies is no longer analogous. Why is it, then, that in that case the fact that the embryo was initially created with the intention to bring a child into the world *does* imply the embryo is treated respectfully?

Jonathan Pugh's analysis of the argument of respect in support of the discarded–created distinction is particularly helpful here. Pugh himself does not support the discarded–created distinction but he tries to reconstruct the respect for the embryo argument in a way that most plausibly could justify the distinction.

Departing from Stephen Darwall's concept of 'recognition respect',[69] Pugh develops the following model of respect:

> it seems that when we claim that something is worthy of moral respect in a given situation, we are stating that there is a morally relevant aspect concerning that thing, or the context of which that thing is part, which ought to bear weight in our moral deliberations . . . In view of this, one reasonable guideline that might be suggested here is that affording proper moral respect to an entity involves setting constraints upon our action that honour or safeguard something that is judged to be morally relevant about the entity in question.[70]

This is very plausible. For example, we could say that in respecting animals, we set constraints upon our behaviour that honour or safeguard the morally relevant property of the animal, for example, the fact that it is sentient. With regard to corpses, we do not honour or safeguard sentience, but something else that we think is morally relevant about corpses.

So what is it that is morally significant about the early embryo? As outlined in Chapter 1, the main reason why people accord an intermediate moral status to the early embryo is that it has the potential to develop into a person. Pugh also believes that this is the most plausible basis to accord an intermediate moral status to the embryo. So, what is morally significant about the embryo is its potential. Let us assume this is true. On the basis of Pugh's model of respect we can derive from this that respectful treatment of the embryo means that we should constrain our actions in a way that honours or safeguards this potential.

It is this, according to Pugh, which can explain why those defending the discarded–created distinction believe that discarded embryos, but not research embryos, are treated with respect. Their belief might be grounded on the fact that

> the intention underlying the creation of SCNT embryos in therapeutic cloning fails to acknowledge the embryo's potential in any way. The attitude that this intention conveys towards the embryo lacks any appreciation of the embryo's

---

[69] Darwall, 'Two Kinds of Respect'.

[70] Jonathan Pugh. 'Is the 'Compromise Position' Concerning the Moral Permissibility of Different Forms of Human Embryonic Stem Cell Research a Tenable Position?', M.Sc. thesis (University of Edinburgh, 2010) and 'Embryos, the Principle of Proportionality, and the Shaky Ground of Moral Respect', *Bioethics* 2013 doi: 10.1111/bioe.12013.

potential. The embryo is never regarded as a potential person, but only as a medical resource; for this reason, this attitude strikes many as particularly exploitative, whilst the intention underlying the creation of the unwanted embryos used in standard hESC research does, albeit to a limited extent.

This also explains why in the passage already quoted FitzPatrick speaks of a 'distinct kind of exploitative attitude' towards research embryos. The idea is that, if embryos are created for reproductive purposes, this acknowledges their potential to become a person and, therefore, treats them with more respect than if they are created for other purposes than reproduction.

But is this sufficient to show that the discarded–created distinction is correct? I believe it is not.

Even if it is true that this explains why discarded embryos are treated with more respect than research embryos, this difference must be so small that it cannot possibly support the discarded–created distinction.

Although the aim of woman-friendly IVF is to create a child, the reason why many more embryos are created than will likely be needed is to prevent or reduce harm to the woman undergoing IVF. Each embryo's chances of developing into a child are significantly reduced by the existence of the other embryos. If one believes this is permissible, given that there is also embryo-friendly IVF, then one cannot accord much moral status to the embryo.

Indeed, FitzPatrick rightly argues that

Even if there is something specially exploitative about research cloning, we must remember what sort of entity we're dealing with. The embryo whose exploitation we are worrying about is something that is at the same time viewed—at least by those who already accept IVF—as possessing a moral status low enough to justify foreseeably sacrificing embryos by the tens of thousands in IVF treatment, and deliberately destroying spares for research.[71]

Pugh comes to the same conclusion: the form of moral respect that is required to be consistent with creating and discarding embryos in IVF must be so diluted that it is hard to see why it cannot be outweighed by the strong moral reasons we have to conduct research using stem cells from research embryos.

Moreover, one may wonder in what way the creation and destruction of research embryos to improve fertility treatments acknowledges

---

[71] FitzPatrick, 'Surplus Embryos', 34.

the potential of the embryo. Those who approve of woman-friendly IVF presumably also approve of research to perfect the IVF technique (for example, by improving methods of *in vitro* culture) or to make it more embryo-friendly (for example, by perfecting techniques to cryo-preserve gametes). This requires research on embryos especially created for the purpose of research.[72] Perhaps the defender of the discarded–created distinction could argue that creating and destroying research embryos to improve assisted reproduction is permissible because it acknowledges the embryos' potential (the research has something to do with reproduction), but it seems to me that this stretches the meaning of 'acknowledging the embryos' potential' a bit too much to be plausible.

To conclude, it seems inconsistent that defenders of the discarded–created distinction are so offended by the idea of the creation and destruction of research embryos as to oppose it despite the enormous expected benefits of the research for a large number of people, while at the same time accepting the creation and destruction of embryos, including of research embryos, in the context of IVF. Only one argument seems to be left to defend this apparently inconsistent position, and that is to show that discarded embryos die in the service of significantly more important goods than research embryos.

Dying in the service of more important goods

Some people may disagree with my claim that stem cell research could produce more or an equal amount of good than the creation of surplus embryos in IVF. They may argue that the goods produced by IVF are more important than the goods produced by research using research embryos. Permissive attitudes to (and regulations regarding) the destructive use of embryos in the context of IVF have mostly been justified by reference to the right to reproductive liberty, which in turn has been justified by pointing to the central position of reproductive projects in people's lives. These justifications cannot be invoked to defend the use of embryos in the context of research.[73]

[72] D. Solter et al., *Embryo Research in Pluralistic Europe* (Berlin and Heidelberg: Springer-Verlag, 2003), 45–52.
[73] Søren Holm, 'The Ethical Case Against Stem Cell Research', *Cambridge Quarterly of Healthcare Ethics*, 12 (2003), 372–83.

Although this is true, it seems implausible that protecting reproductive liberty and helping infertile people to realize their wish for a child produces more important goods than saving people's lives. After all, it is generally accepted that saving lives is more important than creating lives. It is also plausible that saving lives is more important than protecting reproductive liberty. Moreover, that the right to reproductive liberty is a good justification for offering woman-friendly IVF is controversial.

There are other reasons why the goods produced by IVF could be more important. One may argue that by not creating surplus embryos we *harm* women undergoing IVF, whereas by not creating research embryos we merely *allow harm* to occur to individuals in need of stem cell based therapies. As mentioned when discussing the agency cost and the nothing-is-lost principle, many believe that it is typically worse to do harm than to allow harm to occur. For example, many believe that it is typically wrong to kill a person even in circumstances in which it would be permissible to let that person die. However, although it may be true that not creating surplus IVF embryos causes at least some of the harm to women undergoing IVF (as they may have to undergo the hormone treatment and egg retrieval procedure several times), it is mainly the women's decision to proceed with IVF which harms them. Not creating surplus embryos can then be seen as 'merely' allowing harm to occur and consequently is, morally speaking, on a par with not creating research embryos. The 'doing versus allowing harm' distinction, insofar as it has any force in this context, cannot provide a ground for arguing that the goods produced by using discarded IVF embryos are greater than those produced by using research embryos.[74]

---

[74] To support the claim that creating surplus embryos in IVF produces more important goods one may also argue (1) that we should care more about current harms to present individuals than about future harms to them or (2) that we should give more weight to harm to current individuals than to harm to future individuals. (For a defence of the moral distance argument, see e.g. Raziel Abelson, 'Moral Distance: What do we Owe to Unknown Strangers?', *Philosophical Forum*, 36 (2005), 31–9.) However, first, it seems implausible that mere location in time accords special significance to a benefit or harm. Likewise, the fact that the women undergoing IVF exist now does not make the goods produced by destroying embryos for IVF more important than the goods produced by destroying embryos to prevent harm to future persons in need of stem cell-based treatments. For arguments against the moral distance argument, see e.g. Peter Singer, 'Famine, Affluence, and Morality', *Philosophy and Public Affairs*, 1 (1972), 229–43.

2.7. Conclusion

I started by investigating how proponents of the discarded–created distinction justify the derivation of stem cells from discarded embryos and showed that this justification also applies, at least at first sight, to the destruction of research embryos. There are equally strong reasons of beneficence to pursue both types of stem cell research, and we have reasons to believe that both types of research are in accordance with the proportionality principle. This suggested that there should be a presumption against the discarded–created distinction. I then considered whether this presumption can be overridden by investigating the most important arguments adduced in support of the discarded–created distinction. I concluded that these arguments cannot convincingly support the discarded–created distinction. The argument that we should always opt for the least controversial approach and, therefore, should only permit the derivation of stem cells from discarded embryos not only assumes too quickly that this will enable us to achieve the intended research goals, but also begs the question. That destroying research embryos is the most controversial approach is exactly what needs to be argued for. The nothing-is-lost principle cannot justify the discarded–created distinction either. Whether one performs stem cell research using discarded embryos or research embryos, one encourages the creation of embryos that are doomed to be destroyed. The agency cost involved when a researcher destroys a research embryo seems to be equally large as the agency cost involved when a researcher destroys a discarded embryo. Perhaps one could object to my argument that the agency cost involved when a researcher destroys a research embryo is much larger because it is significantly worse to encourage the creation of embryos doomed to die in the context of embryonic stem cell research than it is to encourage the creation of embryos doomed to die in the context of assisted reproduction? If this is true, then the agency cost involved in destroying a research embryo might be too large to be outweighed by the good that is expected to come out of it, even though the agency cost associated with destroying a discarded embryo could be outweighed by the good that is expected to come out of it. This could rescue the nothing-is-lost argument. I considered two arguments that have been adduced to show that it is significantly worse to create and destroy embryos for research than it is to create and destroy embryos in the context of assisted reproduction. A first argument holds that the creation and destruction of discarded embryos can be justified by Double Effect, whereas the creation and destruction of research embryos cannot. However, I argued that, if the embryo is a person, the proportionality condition of Double Effect is not met. The significant harm to embryos is out of proportion to the benefits gained by women undergoing IVF. Only if the embryo has a very low intermediate moral status could the proportionality condition be met, but then the moral status of the embryo must be so low that it becomes very difficult to justify rejecting the creation and destruction of research embryos, given the enormous benefits this could create. The second argument adduced to show that it is significantly worse to create and destroy embryos for research than it is to create and destroy embryos in the context of assisted reproduction refers to the concept of respect. It holds that in the latter case the embryo is treated with respect but not in the former. The argument from respect cannot justify the destruction of an embryo if it is a person and has a right to life. If the embryo has a lower intermediate moral status, however, then perhaps it could. The most plausible interpretation of the argument of respect underlying the discarded–created distinction is that the intention underlying the creation of research embryos fails to acknowledge the embryo's potential in any way. I concluded, however, that even if this can explain there is some moral difference between creating and destroying research embryos and discarded embryos, it cannot explain there is a significant moral difference between these two types of research. This is because the form of moral respect that is required to be consistent with woman-friendly IVF and the destruction of discarded embryos is so diluted that it is hard to see why it cannot be outweighed by the strong moral reasons we have to conduct research using stem cells from research embryos. Moreover, if defenders of the discarded–created distinction think woman-friendly IVF is permissible, presumably they accept the research that is done to develop and improve this technique, and this requires the creation of research embryos.

It seems, then, that once one accepts the derivation of stem cells from discarded embryos, consistency requires that one also accept the derivation of stem cells from research embryos. Since there is a presumption against the discarded–created distinction, we should reject it as an ethical position as long as no better arguments are adduced to support it.

3

The Use–Derivation Distinction

3.1. The Use–Derivation Distinction

In Chapter 2, I argued that, since there is a presumption against the discarded–created distinction and no convincing arguments have been adduced in its defence, we should, for now, regard it as an untenable ethical position. Plausibly, the permissibility of deriving stem cells from embryos is independent of the origin of the embryos; it is either permissible to derive stem cells from both discarded embryos and research embryos, or from neither source. Indeed, another popular middle-ground position in the embryonic stem cell debate holds that deriving stem cells from an embryo is always wrong, regardless of the origin of the embryo. According to this position, while deriving stem cells from an embryo is always wrong, merely using embryonic stem cells may nevertheless be permissible. In this chapter, I investigate whether this middle ground position offers a tenable solution to the Problem.

Most stem cell researchers working with embryonic stem cells do not actually derive the stem cells themselves. The majority only uses embryonic stem cells derived by other researchers, often in other countries. Some have argued that, even if the derivation of stem cells from an early embryo is always wrong because it destroys the embryo, it may be permissible to conduct research on embryonic stem cells that were derived by others. I will refer to the middle-ground position that draws a moral line between the use and the derivation of embryonic stem cells as

The Use–Derivation Distinction. It is presumptively permissible to use embryonic stem cells in research, even though it is always impermissible to derive embryonic stem cells.

Stem cell policies in several countries and jurisdictions, including in Italy, Germany, and the United States, are based on the use–derivation distinction. In Germany, for example, it is illegal for researchers to derive stem cells from embryos, but research with embryonic stem cells that were imported from abroad is, under certain conditions, permitted.

Before I proceed to discussing the arguments adduced in support of the use–derivation distinction, let me first comment on an assumption underlying this middle-ground position.

3.2. The Moral Status of Embryonic Stem Cells

A necessary assumption for accepting the use–derivation distinction is that embryonic stem cells are not themselves embryos, nor their moral equivalents. If they were, then 'merely' using embryonic stem cells in research would be tantamount to destructive embryo research, which defenders of the use–derivation distinction reject.

Embryonic stem cells are not embryos

That embryonic stem cells are not embryos, or their moral equivalents, is typically taken for granted; it is not normally explicitly stated. In the US, however, the explicit claim that embryonic stem cells are not embryos has played a crucial role in the development of federal stem cell policy regarding embryonic stem cell research. In the US, restrictions on research using embryos are largely confined to federal funding limitations. Federal support for research involving the destruction of human embryos has been banned since the 1970s. An attempt by President Clinton to partly remove the ban and allow federal funding of research using discarded embryos was blocked when, in 1995 Congress passed a bill along with a rider called the Dickey-Wicker Amendment. This amendment prohibits the Department of Health and Human Services (HHS) from using federal money for research 'in which a human embryo or embryos are destroyed, discarded, or knowingly subjected to risk of injury or death greater than allowed for research on foetuses *in utero*'.[1] HHS funds the National Institutes of Health (NIH), the primary agency of the government responsible for biomedical and health-related

---

[1]   Congress, t. 1995 H. R. 2127; 1404 H. R. 2127. C. o. A. House of Representatives (1995).

research. Thus, since the Dickey-Wicker Amendment was passed, research that may harm embryos has not been federally funded. When the Dickey-Wicker Amendment was written in 1995, it was not introduced with human embryonic stem cell research in mind, as no such research had yet been done. James Thomson's laboratory first reported the isolation of embryonic stem cells from human embryos in 1998. This research was supported by private money. In 1999, in an attempt to enable federal funding for at least some embryonic stem cell research, the General Counsel of HHS, Harriet Rabb, wrote in a legal opinion that the restrictions of the Dickey-Wicker Amendment 'would not apply to research utilizing human pluripotent stem cells because such cells are not a human embryo within the statutory definition'.[2] Rabb claimed that 'a human embryo, as that term is virtually universally understood, has the potential to develop in the normal course of events into a living human being', and that pluripotent stem cells do not have this capacity. Rabb concluded that federal funding involving research *using* stem cells derived from embryos was 'lawful, so long as private funds were used to derive the cells from the embryos'. Rabb thus introduced the use–derivation distinction. It was subsequently accepted, though with different qualifications, by the Clinton, Bush, and Obama administrations. No federal money would be used to support the derivation of embryonic stem cells, as that would violate the Dickey-Wicker Amendment. However, federal money could be used, under certain conditions, for research using embryonic stem cells derived with private money, or abroad.

Let us now consider the arguments underlying the claim that embryonic stem cells are not embryos. Rabb's first argument, that embryonic stem cells are not embryos because they are not embryos within the statutory definition, though legally important, is not helpful for determining whether embryonic stem cells are *actually* embryos, or their moral equivalents. It does not follow from the fact that embryonic stem cells are not included within the legal definition of an embryo that they *should* not be included. Even if embryonic stem cells are not legally embryos they might still be embryos from a biological point of view, or they might have the same moral status as embryos. It may turn out, for example, that the moral status of embryonic stem cells is equal or

² Harriet S. Rabb, letter to H. Varmus (NIH), 'Federal Funding for Research Involving Human Pluripotent Stem Cells' (General Council, Washington, DC, 15 Jan. 1999).

very similar to that of embryos, and this could provide a reason to include them in the legal definition of an embryo. Before the birth of Dolly the cloned sheep, an embryo-like organism created through cloning was not part of any definition of an embryo. But after ethical debate it was determined that we have good reason to include such an organism in the legal definition of an embryo. Many agreed that an embryo-like cell or cluster of cells produced through cloning has the same morally relevant characteristics, and thus the same moral status, as an embryo resulting from the fusion of a sperm cell and an oocyte. Perhaps we may also conclude after ethical debate that embryonic stem cells share the morally relevant characteristics of an embryo, and therefore should legally be considered an embryo. A good place to start such an ethical debate is Rabb's second argument in defence of the claim that embryonic stem cells are not embryos. Rabb states that, unlike embryos, embryonic stem cells lack the potential to develop, in the normal course of events, into a living human being. As mentioned in Chapters 1 and 2, it is very common to accord a significant moral status to the embryo in virtue of its potential to develop into a person, or in virtue of a valuable future that this potential makes possible.[3] The argument underlying the claim that the embryo derives its significant moral status from this potential is generally referred to as 'the potentiality argument'. In the next section, I argue that if the potentiality argument in defence of the embryo's significant moral status is correct, then we may also have to accord a significant moral status to embryonic stem cells, as there is reason to believe that they too have the potential to develop into persons. If embryonic stem cells could be regarded as potential persons, opponents of the derivation of embryonic stem cells who adhere to the potentiality argument are faced with an interesting dilemma: they must either treat embryonic stem cells as morally significant entities worthy of protection and thus oppose the use of embryonic stem cells, or admit that early embryos do not derive their significant moral status from the potential they possess. Either way, unless they can find another convincing reason to accord a significant moral status to the embryo, they will have to reject the use–derivation distinction.

[3] Don Marquis, 'Why Abortion is Immoral', *Journal of Philosophy*, 86 (1989), 183–202.

Are embryonic stem cells potential babies?

If the human embryo has the potential to become a person and is supposedly morally important in virtue of that potential, then every other cell or organism with the same or a very similar potential must be assigned equal moral importance. This argument has sometimes been referred to as 'the (absurd) extension argument'.[4] The extension argument has been adduced to show that since oocytes and sperm put together in a petri dish also have the potential to develop into a person, they should be accorded a significant moral status too.[5] Since the possibility of SCNT in mammals, some have also argued that each mammalian body cell has the potential to become a person.[6] If these extension arguments are correct, then this has absurd implications for the potentiality argument. Our body would consist of millions of potential persons, and we would have to protect each one of them!

In what follows, I apply the extension argument to embryonic stem cells.[7] I argue that scientific experiments suggest that embryonic stem cells may have a potential that is similar enough to that of the embryo to cast doubt on the claim that embryonic stem cells have no significant moral status (assuming the potentiality argument is correct). The debate on the potentiality argument is a wide-ranging one. I restrict myself here

---

[4] David B. Annis, 'Abortion and the Potentiality Principle', *Southern Journal of Philosophy*, 22 (1984), 155–63. Marco Stier and Bettina Schoene-Seifert, 'The Argument from Potentiality in the Embryo Protection Debate: Finally "Depotentialized"?', *American Journal of Bioethics*, 13 (2013), 19–27.

[5] L. W. Sumner, *Abortion and Moral Theory* (Princeton: Princeton University Press, 1981). Helga Kuhse and Peter Singer, 'The Moral Status of the Embryo', in William A. W. Walters and Peter Singer (eds), *Test-Tube Babies: A Guide to Moral Questions, Present Techniques, and Future Possibilities* (Melbourne: Oxford University Press, 1982), 57–63. Peter Singer and Karen Dawson, 'IVF Technology and the Argument from Potential', *Philosophy and Public Affairs*, 17 (1988), 90.

[6] See e.g. Julian Savulescu, 'Should we Clone Human Beings? Cloning as a Source of Tissue for Transplantation', *Journal of Medical Ethics*, 25 (1999), 87–95. Alta R. Charo, 'Every Cell is Sacred', in Paul Lauritzen (ed.), *Cloning and the Future of Human Embryo Research* (Oxford: Oxford University Press, 2001), 82–9. Gerard Magill and William B. Neaves, 'Ontological and Ethical Implications of Direct Nuclear Reprogramming', *Kennedy Institute of Ethics Journal*, 19 (2009), 23–32.

[7] This section is partly based on Katrien Devolder and Christopher M. Ward, 'Rescuing Human Embryonic Stem Cell Research: The Possibility of Embryo Reconstitution', *Metaphilosophy*, 28 (2007), 245–63, and Katrien Devolder, 'To Be, or Not to Be?', *EMBO Reports*, 10 (2009), 1285–7.

to briefly discussing the most important arguments that have been adduced in the embryonic stem cell debate.

Tetraploid complementation

The thought that embryonic stem cells may have very similar potential to that of an embryo is suggested by a technique called 'tetraploid complementation'. This technique shows that embryonic stem cells can give rise to a live-born organism when provided with a surrogate trophectoderm (which forms the placenta and the membranes that nourish and protect the developing organism in the uterus).

Tetraploid complementation is a process normally used to test the pluripotency of stem cells and has been used routinely in the mouse. The technique involves creating tetraploid embryos by fusing the cells (blastomeres) of two-cell stage embryos by exposing them to an electric current. The resulting one-cell tetraploid embryos will have twice the normal of chromosomes (four sets, instead of two, hence the term 'tetraploid'). These cells will then begin to divide and all daughter cells will also be tetraploid. Because each cell in such tetraploid embryos has twice the normal number of chromosomes, these embryos do not result in life offspring when transferred to the uterus. However, when mouse embryonic stem cells are injected into the tetraploid embryos, either at the morula (16–32 cells) or at the blastocyst stage (125–250 cells) stage, and the resulting organism is implanted in the uterus of a surrogate mouse, a normal mouse embryo and foetus develops. What is striking about this technique is that the resulting mouse pups are derived *solely* from the embryonic stem cells, which means that the tetraploid embryos *only* acted as a substitute trophectoderm, which forms the placenta and other nourishing membranes but which does not contribute to the 'embryo proper' (which will eventually become the live-born organism).[8]

Thus, what tetraploid complementation experiments in the mouse show is that embryonic stem cells can, when injected into a tetraploid embryo, give rise to an entire organism. Ethical issues prevent these experiments from being carried out in humans as scientists would have to let the embryos that they have created develop to term. However, despite differences in human and mouse stem cell populations, several

---

[8] Andras Nagy et al., 'Embryonic Stem Cells Alone are Able to Support Foetal Development in the Mouse', *Development*, 110 (1990), 815–21.

scientists have stated that it is reasonable to assume that human embryonic stem cells might have the same potential as mouse embryonic stem cells.[9] That is to say, *if* human embryonic stem cells were injected into human tetraploid embryos, that are subsequently transferred to a woman's uterus, they might give rise to a live-born human infant, and ultimately an adult human being.

We could conclude from this that embryonic stem cells are likely to be potential persons and, thus, should be treated accordingly. Developmental biologist, Hans Werner Denker, is probably the most ardent defender of this view. Denker writes that,

[a]lthough experiments in the mouse show that the efficiency of cloning by tetraploid complementation depends on the particular mouse strain from which the embryonic stem cells were derived, we must, by extrapolation, regard embryonic stem cells in humans basically as potential human beings as long as it has not been shown that the respective cell line cannot form an embryo by tetraploid complementation.[10]

Denker takes it to follow from this view that embryonic stem cells have a significant moral and legal status. It might seem that, for those who accord a significant moral status to the early embryo in virtue of its potential to become a person, the results of tetraploid complementation raise the interesting dilemma mentioned above: those who adopt this view must either treat embryonic stem cells as morally significant entities worthy of protection and thus oppose the use of embryonic stem cells, or admit that early embryos do not derive their significant moral status from the potential they possess, and thus reject the potentiality argument.

There may, however, be a way out of this dilemma. One could argue that, despite the capacity of embryonic stem cells to give rise to live-born humans via tetraploid complementation, they nevertheless lack some morally significant kind of potential that embryos possess.

The need for a surrogate trophoblast

The most obvious argument to demonstrate the moral difference between the potential of embryonic stem cells and that of embryos is

---

[9] See e.g. H. W. Denker, 'Potentiality of Embryonic Stem Cells: An Ethical Problem Even with Alternative Stem Cell Sources', *Journal of Medical Ethics*, 32 (2006), 665–71. Wenlin Li et al., 'Generation of Rat and Human Induced Pluripotent Stem Cells by Combining Genetic Reprogramming and Chemical Inhibitors', *Cell Stem Cell*, 4 (2009), 16–19.

[10] Denker, 'Potentiality of Embryonic Stem Cells', 669.

that embryonic stem cells *alone* cannot give rise to a full-grown organism. Whereas embryos have the capacity to produce their own trophoblast, which is essential for embryonic development, embryonic stem cells require the provision of a *surrogate* trophoblast by tetraploid embryos.[11]

Although this observation is accurate, it is not clear that it is morally relevant. An ordinary blastocyst consists of two distinct cell types: inner cell mass (ICM) cells, which become the embryo proper and, eventually, the adult organism; and trophoblast cells, which contribute to the placental support system. Although the trophoblast is essential for the development of the embryo, it does not become part of the embryo proper and, thus, of the full-grown organism. Arguably, then, it is the ICM cells that are of moral significance, as the trophoblast merely provides the appropriate environment for these cells to develop into the embryo.

Consider the following hypothetical case:

Defective Trophoblast. A couple undergoing IVF can only produce embryos with a defective trophoblast. These embryos are unlikely to develop into a healthy baby. Fortunately, tetraploid complementation with human cells has become a routine technique. The defective trophoblast of each of the couple's embryos can be replaced with a surrogate trophoblast. To circumvent the moral issue of destroying embryos to provide such a surrogate trophoblast it is not made from embryos.[12] When the embryos with the defective trophoblast reach the blastocyst stage, their inner cell masses are isolated and injected into the surrogate trophoblasts. The inner cell mass cells survive the procedure and when transferred to the uterus along with the new trophoblasts, can result in a successful pregnancy.

---

[11] This argument has been adduced to show that gametes or somatic cells have a different kind of potential compared to embryos. See e.g. Alfonso Gómez-Lobo, 'Does Respect for Embryos Entail Respect for Gametes?', *Theoretical Medicine and Bioethics*, 25 (2004), 202.

[12] Recall that to create a surrogate trophectoderm via tetraploid complementation, cells of two-cell-staged embryos need to be fused. This could be considered problematic for those who accord a significant moral status to the embryo. But a possible solution to this problem could be to use embryonic stem cell-derived trophoblast cells. Scientific evidence suggests that embryonic stem cells can differentiate into trophoblast lineages. Behzad Gerami-Naini et al., 'Trophoblast Differentiation in Embryoid Bodies Derived from Human Embryonic Stem Cells', *Endocrinology*, 145 (2004), 1517–24. R. Harun et al., 'Cytotrophoblast Stem Cell Lines Derived from Human Embryonic Stem Cells and their Capacity to Mimic Invasive Implantation Events', *Human Reproduction*, 21 (2006), 1349–58.

Would those who think that potential is what determines the moral status of the embryo object to applying this technique to fulfil the couple's wish for a child? Probably not. Yet, the structure of the full embryo—ICM plus (defective) trophoblast—is compromised. If it is really potential what matters, then it seems that it is not the embryo as a whole that should merit special protection, but the cell or cells that can actually give rise to a child. Suppose we are in the middle of the tetraploid complementation procedure. We have isolated the ICM and are about to inject it in the surrogate trophoblast. Presumably most who accord a significant moral status to the embryo will think that the entity in the middle of the procedure has the same moral status as the embryo, even though the entity lacks the potential to develop into a child without the external addition of a trophoblast. If the ICM merits special protection in this scenario, then embryonic stem cells too should merit special protection as they have the same potential to give rise to a full-grown organism. ICM cells and embryonic stem cells can both develop into a full-grown organism but both require a surrogate trophoblast or another suitable substitute to do so.

The fact that the trophoblast and the embryonic stem cells or ICM cells are in constant interaction, and that the latter need nutrients and signals from the former to develop further, does not make it less plausible that embryonic stem cells and ICM cells have similar enough potential to that of an embryo to demand similar treatment. After all, the development of a cell or cells *always* depends on interaction with a context. This is as true for embryonic stem cells as it is for zygotes (fertilized oocytes) and embryonic cells. A cell, or group of cells, can exist in many states in the body or in the laboratory, depending on what sort of information it receives. To develop into a foetus and a full-grown human being, an early embryo must implant in the uterus and communicate and interact with neighbouring cells, the extracellular matrix and the blood or lymph, and must not be exposed to dangerous substances. Likewise, the development of embryonic stem cells into a foetus and full-grown organism depends on continuous interaction with a similarly supportive environment.[13] The fact that this environment is provided by researchers is morally irrelevant, as this is also the case with embryos *in vitro* created via

---

[13] This has been pointed out many times before, e.g. in Singer and Dawson, 'IVF Technology'.

IVF. These embryos need to be implanted into a uterus to further develop. Yet proponents of the potentiality argument think that IVF embryos have the kind of potential that matters for moral status.

Active and passive potential

One could still object that, unlike embryonic stem cells, an embryo, whether produced through IVF or sexual reproduction, has some sort of 'force' *inside* it that determines what it will become. The context or environment merely allows the expression of the embryo's potential. With embryonic stem cells, by contrast, it might seem that it is the *external* manipulations (for example, provision of a tetraploid tropho-blast) that are really determining what sort of thing the cells will give rise to. The first type of potential is typically referred to as 'intrinsic' or 'active', the second type—supposedly possessed by embryonic stem cells—as 'extrinsic' or 'passive'.[14] Aristotle made the distinction between these two types of potential in his discussion of potentiality in *The Metaphysics*. The typical example used to illustrate the different poten-tials is that of a conker and a horse chestnut tree. To become a horse chestnut tree, a conker just needs 'appropriate circumstances', but for the tree to be turned into a table, an external agent—a carpenter—is needed.[15] Thus, the conker has intrinsic or active potential to become a tree, but the tree has only extrinsic or passive potential to become a table. It could be argued that only entities with *intrinsic* or *active* potential to become persons have a significant moral status and should not be des-troyed for research. It must then also be shown that embryos have active potential, whereas embryonic stem cells merely have passive potential.

Maureen Condic, Patrick Lee, and Robert George—influential critics of the extension argument—appeal to the distinction between active and passive potential when criticizing Gerard Magill and William Neaves, who also claim that embryonic stem cells have the potential to become a person. They write that

---

[14] See e.g. the US Conference of Catholic Bishops write about an embryo that '[a]s a matter of biological fact, this new living organism has the full complement of human genes and is actively expressing those genes to live and develop in a way that is unique to human beings, setting the essential foundation for further development'. *On Embryonic Stem Cell Research: A Statement of the United States Conference of Catholic Bishops*, 2008. <http://stemcell.www65.a2hosting.com/wp-content/uploads/2013/11/usccb_2008-06-13.pdf>.

[15] Stephen Holland, *Bioethics: A Philosophical Introduction* (Oxford: Polity, 2002).

[s]imply because a house can be converted into a pile of rubble by the action of a tornado does not in any way eliminate the important differences between a house and a pile of rubble. Thus, Magill and Neaves make a fundamental logical error in confusing what a cell can be converted into by a technological intervention— what in philosophical terms is called the 'passive potency' of the cell, that is, the susceptibility of the cell to be transformed by the actions upon it of extrinsic agents—with what the cell actually is, which is determined by its active potency for self-development.[16]

This argument has been adduced against previous applications of the extension argument. For example, it has been said that oocytes and sperm only contain active potential after being fused together; before such fusion they have only passive potential and thus lack the special moral status of a zygote or embryo. Helen Watt, for example, writes that

[w]hat the unfertilised, unactivated ovum does not have is the active potential to develop as an organism. This is shown by the fact that no development takes place until what begins as the interior of the ovum receives the contents of the sperm. . . . while the ovum has, as a whole, the passive potential to be turned into part of the zygote, this is not a kind of passive potential which is compatible with its survival.[17]

In similar vein, it has been argued that only the cell resulting from nuclear transfer—that is, *after* the somatic cell has been fused with an enucleated egg—has active potential. Only after this event does a new cell exist that 'has the right dynamic' to give rise to live offspring.

However, even if the distinction between extrinsic and intrinsic potential is morally significant in the cases just described, it is not clear that it can be used to justify assigning a lower moral status to embryonic stem cells than to embryos. An embryo can be created entirely from embryonic stem cells by simply transferring them into an appropriate environment—unlike with SCNT or gametes, no new cell needs to be created. It would be similar to placing a conker in fertile soil. Thus, it seems that an embryonic stem cell has the intrinsic potential to become an embryo and thus a person (at least, in the same sense that an embryo *in vitro* has the intrinsic potential to become a person).

[16] Maureen L. Condic, Patrick Lee, and Robert P. George, 'Ontological and Ethical Implications of Direct Nuclear Reprogramming: Response to Magill and Neaves', *Kennedy Institute of Ethics Journal*, 19 (2009), 34.

[17] Helen Watt, 'Potential and the Early Human', *Journal of Medical Ethics*, 22 (1996), 223.

The use–derivation distinction under pressure

The assumption that embryonic stem cells are neither embryos nor their moral equivalents should not be taken for granted by those who accord a significant moral status to the embryo in virtue of its potential to become a person. Although embryonic stem cells and embryos may not be identical in their potential to develop into a person, both have the capacity, at least in theory, to develop into a person when placed in an appropriate environment. Those who oppose the derivation of embryonic stem cells because it kills potential persons must find a more convincing way of distinguishing the potential of embryonic stem cells and embryos. If they cannot do so, they must either oppose the use of embryonic stem cells too (and thus reject the use–derivation distinction), or they must reject the potentiality argument, and eschew restrictions on the derivation of embryonic stem cells, or seek some other basis for them. Of course, this dilemma does not necessarily exist for those who accord a significant moral status to the embryo on grounds independent of their potential. Thus, my argument does not cast doubt on their defence of the use–derivation distinction. So let us now turn to the arguments adduced in support of this distinction. How convincing are they?

3.3. Benefiting from Others' Wrongdoing

The use–derivation distinction holds that using embryonic stem cells in research may be permissible even if it is always impermissible to derive embryonic stem cells. An important question that arises and that proponents of the use–derivation distinction must answer is: how can it be permissible to make use of cellular products that were obtained through a putatively impermissible act? True, those who merely use embryonic stem cells do not themselves destroy embryos. They do, however, benefit from earlier embryo destruction performed by others, and most agree that benefiting from others' wrongdoing is typically wrong itself. For example, the production of child pornography is wrong, and so is benefiting from it (for example, by purchasing or watching it). Defenders of the use–derivation distinction will thus have to explain why it is not wrong to use embryonic stem cells, even though this involves benefiting from embryo destruction. Before turning to their arguments, I should say something more about why it is that benefiting from others' wrongdoing may be wrong itself.

Encouraging wrongdoing

One reason why it is sometimes wrong to benefit from others' wrongdoing is that this will encourage further wrongdoing. In section 2.4, I argued that when a researcher derives stem cells from an embryo, she not only causes the loss of the current embryo's (valuable) life, she also encourages similar losses in the future. The researcher benefits from woman-friendly IVF practices, or from the creation of research embryos by others, and either way she thereby encourages the repetition of the sort of wrongdoing involved in these practices.

Most agree that encouraging others' wrongdoing is presumptively wrong—it is wrong, unless special circumstances obtain that justify it (for example, if encouraging someone to kill an innocent person is the only way to prevent a thousand innocent persons from being killed). There are several ways in which one may encourage others' wrongdoing. Ronald Green's distinctions are helpful here.[18] Green distinguishes between

(1) *Direct encouragement of the wrong act through agency.* This sort of encouragement occurs when someone knowingly and intentionally uses an agent to commit a wrong. For example, Bob hires an assassin to kill Jeff. This sort of encouragement could take place in embryonic stem cell research if a researcher who wants to use embryonic stem cells explicitly asks another researcher to derive these cells for him.

(2) *Direct encouragement through the acceptance of benefit.* For this sort of encouragement, no direct agency relationship needs to exist. Bob commits a wrong independently of Jeff but Jeff receives some benefit from Bob's wrongdoing. Instead of punishing Bob or at least condemning his act, Jeff accepts the benefits. This encourages Bob to repeat the wrongdoing. This sort of encouragement could take place in embryonic stem cell research if a researcher, by using embryonic stem cells derived by others (but not on her command), directly encourages these 'others' to derive more embryonic stem cells.

---

[18] Ronald M. Green, 'Benefiting from "Evil": An Incipient Moral Problem in Human Stem Cell Research', *Bioethics*, 16 (2002), 544–56.

(3) *Indirect encouragement through legitimization of a practice*. In this case it is not the immediate impact of one's acceptance of the benefit on identifiable wrongdoers that matters. Central here is the future impact on people generally of 'the public rule of conduct' that is created by one's acceptance of the benefits of wrongdoing. What Green has in mind is that benefiting from others' wrongdoing may result in a more *general acceptance* of that wrongdoing, or similar instances of it. It may, for example, foster more permissive social attitudes towards it, thereby increasing the likelihood of it reoccurring. In section 2.4, I argued that, by destroying discarded embryos, a researcher may indirectly encourage further embryo destruction by softening social attitudes towards it. Green uses an example outside of the domain of stem cell research to illustrate the idea of indirect encouragement through legitimization of a practice. He refers to the beneficial use of 'medical' data obtained by Nazi doctors during the Second World War through cruel experiments on concentration camp inmates. Why should present-day doctors not use these data in important biomedical research or to inform clinical practice? After all, they cannot, through the use of these data, encourage the Nazi doctors to commit their atrocities again. However, the problem here is that, by using these data, doctors would seem to implicitly condone a morally repellent practice and establish and legitimize a rule that, as long as it benefits other people and cannot encourage the original wrongdoers to repeat their wrongdoing, it is permissible for researchers to use data obtained by research in which innocent individuals are harmed and killed. This rule could send the message to current researchers that their data will be used even if obtained through immoral means, which in turn could lead some researchers to ignore ethical standards of human subject research.

Not all cases of benefiting from others' wrongdoing involve encouraging future instances of the same type of wrongdoing. When we enjoy the beauty of Pyramids built by slaves, we do not encourage slavery, though we benefit from past slavery. Another example is the murder victim case discussed in section 2.4:

> *Murder Victim.* A teen has been murdered in gang violence. After having received consent of the teen's parents, a surgeon uses the murder victim's organs for transplantation to a patient who requires them in order to survive.

Even though the surgeon's action involves benefiting from others' wrongdoing (murder), most would agree that what the surgeon does is permissible. Perhaps this is because we find it very unlikely that, by benefiting from murder, the surgeon encourages further murders in any way. She does not create a demand for murders, nor does she express support for those who murdered the victim or for murder in general. Her intentions are entirely unrelated and in some ways diametrically opposed to those of the murderers (she intends to *save* lives).

Taint and disrespect

There may be other reasons why benefiting from others' wrongdoing can be wrong—reasons independent of the *effects* of one's actions on future wrongdoing. For example, some think that benefiting from wrongdoing may be wrong because being so closely connected to others' wrongdoing brings one 'in touch with evil' or calls one's character into question. One becomes 'tainted' by the wrongdoing of others. Suppose a friend inherits a big sum of money from her deceased grandmother. She knows her grandmother got so rich because she robbed some people in a home for the elderly, but nevertheless accepts the inheritance. One may feel repulsed by her accepting the 'tainted' money and may call her character into question. Another reason why one may disapprove of her accepting the money is that she thereby expresses disrespect for the victims of her grandmother's wrongdoing.

The suggestion that benefiting from others' wrongdoing can be wrong even where it does not encourage future wrongdoing is somewhat controversial.[19] Most agree, however, that benefiting from others' wrongdoing can be wrong when and because it encourages future wrongdoing. Therefore, defenders of the use–derivation distinction have seen it as an important task to show that by using embryonic stem cells, a researcher does not encourage embryo destruction. In fact, this is the main argument in defence of the use–derivation distinction. In the next section, I argue that the use of embryonic stem cells always encourages embryo destruction in a way that makes it presumptively wrong.[20]

[19] John A. Robertson, 'Causative vs. Beneficial Complicity in the Embryonic Stem Cell Debate', *Connecticut Law Review*, 36 (2003), 1099–113. Green, 'Benefiting from Evil'.

[20] I do not mean to say that the fact that something is controversial is a good reason to *not* give it philosophical attention. The reason why I am not going deeper into the issue of

3.4. Using Embryonic Stem Cells and Encouraging Embryo Destruction

In an article, 'Stem Cell Research in a Catholic Institution: Yes or No?', a group of ten authors argues that it is permissible for researchers in a Catholic institution to conduct research with embryonic stem cells as long as these cells were derived (1) from discarded embryos, (2) by others, and (3) not on their request. Making use of stem cells from a stem cell bank would, for example, fit these conditions. The idea is that, when these conditions are met, a researcher using embryonic stem cells does not encourage embryo destruction as

the stem cell lines are going to be available with or without the agreement of Catholic research institutions, and their cooperation is not necessary for the destruction of the embryos to occur.[21]

John Robertson, in defending the use–derivation distinction, has adduced a similar argument. According to Robertson

the claim that benefitting from a past wrong is likely to encourage future instances of that wrong is more difficult to sustain if, as in the case of ES cell derivation, what is perceived as 'wrong' is legally permitted and will occur on a widespread basis whatever the decision of a particular jurisdiction. Because there is or will be sufficient demand from researchers or clinicians to derive new ES cell lines, that derivation is very likely to occur regardless of United States or German policy against derivation. A strong case for banning any support of research and therapy because of its likelihood of encouraging future destruction of embryos cannot easily be made.[22]

Robertson acknowledges that support for the use of embryonic stem cells would contribute to embryonic stem cell research in general, and thus indirectly encourage future embryonic stem cell derivation. But the key question, according to Robertson, is whether such support 'will lead to a significant increase in the destruction of embryos, beyond the number

whether benefiting from others' wrongdoing may be wrong regardless of the effects, is that if I can show that using embryonic stem cells involves encouraging embryo destruction, I have provided sufficient evidence against the use-derivation distinction.

[21] Michael R. Prieur et al., 'Stem Cell Research in a Catholic Institution: Yes or No?', *Kennedy Institute of Ethics Journal*, 16 (2006), 87.

[22] Robertson, 'Causative vs. Beneficial Complicity', 1105–6.

that would have been destroyed', that is, in the absence of such support.[23]

So one argument in support of the use–derivation distinction seems to hold that embryonic stem cell use is permissible if it does not result in an increase, or according to Robertson, a *significant* increase, in the number of embryos destroyed (compared to the number that would have been destroyed had the embryonic stem cell use not occurred). It is assumed that such an increase will not occur, as researchers working in jurisdictions with more permissible stem cell policies create a sufficient demand for embryonic stem cell lines for a large enough supply to be available in any case. Thus, the idea is that, since there will always be a large supply of embryonic stem cell lines for scientists in less restrictive countries, research on embryonic stem cells in restrictive countries will not have an impact on the number of embryos destroyed.

Two questions arise: (1) is it true that by merely using embryonic stem cells, a researcher in a country with a restrictive stem cell policy does not have an effect on the total number of embryos destroyed? And (2) even if this were true, would it be sufficient to show that the mere use of embryonic stem cells does not encourage embryo destruction in a way that makes it presumptively wrong? I start with the first question and argue that a researcher using embryonic stem cells *does* increase the number of embryos destroyed, or can be expected to do so. I then argue that, even if it turns out that by merely *using* embryonic stem cells the researcher definitely did *not* increase the number of embryos destroyed, she may still have encouraged embryo destruction in a way that makes it presumptively wrong.

Increasing the number of embryos destroyed

The main argument for the view that there will *not* be an increase in the number of embryos destroyed by merely using embryonic stem cells is that there currently is a sufficient demand for such cells and an extra user will not increase the supply. Is this a plausible argument?

Consider an anecdote discussed by Peter Singer in defence of vegetarianism.[24] At a conference dinner Singer was sitting opposite a Buddhist philosopher from Thailand. At the buffet, Singer, arguably the most

[23] Robertson, 'Causative vs. Beneficial Complicity', 1106.
[24] Peter Singer, 'A Vegetarian Philosophy', in Sian Griffiths and Jennifer Wallace (eds), *Consuming Passions* (Manchester: Manchester University Press, 1998), 66–72.

famous vegetarian in the world, avoided the meat dishes, but the Buddhist did not. Singer asked him how he reconciled eating meat with the first precept of Buddhist tradition, which tells us to avoid harming sentient beings. The man told Singer that in the Buddhist tradition it is wrong to eat meat only if you have reason to believe that the animal was killed especially for you. The meat he had taken, however, was not from animals killed especially for him; the animal would have died anyway. Hence, by eating it, he was not harming any animals.

The same sort of reasoning as that of the Buddhist has been used to defend the use of already existing embryonic stem cells that were not produced on request. The idea is that the embryonic stem cells used by the researcher were not derived especially for him, and would have been derived anyway because of other researchers creating a sufficient demand for them. Hence, by merely using embryonic stem cells, a researcher is not harming any embryos.

However, Singer rightly points out that the obvious flaw in the Buddhist's argument is that he entirely ignores the rather obvious link between meat consumption and the future killing of animals. Singer writes:

Granted, the chicken lying in the supermarket freezer today would have died even if I had never existed; but the fact that I take the chicken from the freezer, and ignore the tofu on a nearby shelf, has something to do with the number of chickens, or blocks of tofu, the supermarket will order next week and thus contributes, in a small way, to the future growth or decline of the chicken and tofu industries. That is what the laws of supply and demand are all about.[25]

Can we expect that, through the same mechanism of supply and demand, an individual researcher's use of embryonic stem cells will affect the supply of embryonic stem cell lines, and thus the number of embryos destroyed?

There is an obvious disanalogy between the two cases. Embryonic stem cells can proliferate for a very long time (in theory, indefinitely). Thus, an embryonic stem cell line can continuously replenish itself. However, a chicken obviously cannot regenerate. It seems then that when we buy or consume a chicken, we contribute to a demand for more chickens, which

---

[25] Singer, 'Vegetarian Philosophy'.

is likely to result in more chickens being slaughtered.[26] When a researcher uses existing embryonic stem cells, this does not necessarily result in more embryo destruction, as the stem cell line from which the stem cells originate can simply replenish itself, obviating the need to create a new stem cell line.

However, this dissimilarity between the two cases does not mean that *no* mechanism of supply and demand is at work when a researcher uses embryonic stem cells. The mechanism of supply and demand at work is the following: as more and more research groups make progress in embryonic stem cell research, an increasing number of research groups will conduct embryonic stem cell research. This will tend to lead to a diversification in the goals the stem cell researchers seek to realize (more stem cell research will tend to result in a wider variety of stem cell research projects). In addition, progress in some areas of embryonic stem cell research will increase the potential payoffs in other areas of embryonic stem cell research, because of significant complementarities between different types of embryonic stem cell research. This will thus incentivize the further diversification of goals that researchers seek to realize through stem cell research. To achieve these different goals, different kinds of embryonic stem cells will be needed. For example, some researchers may come to need 'safe' stem cells that were not cultured on mouse feeder cells, stem cells containing certain diseases, stem cells that enable the *in vitro* study of that disease, and stem cells genetically identical to the patient. This will result in the creation of new embryonic stem cell lines, and, thus, in more embryo destruction. Empirical research by McCormick, Owen-Smith, and Scott suggests that, such effects have indeed occurred.[27] They researched the number of vials with embryonic stem cell lines distributed within the US between 2000 and 2007, and showed that this number increased significantly over time. Initially, only 'existing stem cell lines' were shipped, but from 2003

---

[26] The mechanism via which this may occur is, however, not straightforward, as the supermarket will normally not order a new chicken each time a chicken is sold. It is typically only when a certain threshold is reached (e.g. the 25th chicken is sold) that the shopkeeper might order new chickens. Thus, an individual who buys the 20th chicken might not have any perceptible effect on the demand for chickens. Shelly Kagan, 'Do I Make a Difference?', *Philosophy and Public Affairs*, 39 (2011), 105–41.

[27] Jennifer B. McCormick, Jason Owen-Smith, and Christopher Thomas Scott, 'Distribution of Human Embryonic Stem Cell Lines: Who, When, and Where', *Cell Stem Cell*, 4 (2009), 107–10.

onwards, newly created embryonic stem cell lines were increasingly shipped (over a four-year period more newly created embryonic stem cell lines were shipped than existing stem cell lines over an eight-year period). An increasing number of laboratories also started to create their own embryonic stem cell lines with private money. The authors conclude that 'despite a patchwork of policies, states with a wide range of federally supported biomedical research contribute to the demand for lines'.[28] This strongly suggests that the 'mere' use of embryonic stem cells does in fact create a demand for more embryonic stem cell lines, and thus encourages embryo destruction.

Another way in which using embryonic stem cells may have an effect on the supply of embryonic stem cell lines is through altering social attitudes towards embryo destruction. In section 2.4, I argued that, by destroying discarded embryos, a researcher may foster permissive social attitudes towards embryo destruction. She would indirectly encourage embryo destruction in the ways described in Green's third type of encouragement, through 'legitimization of a practice'. I think that the same type of encouragement occurs when a researcher merely *uses* embryonic stem cells. Recall Gillam's explanation for why foetal tissue research is likely to indirectly encourage abortion, but why the surgeon's use of a murder victim's organs is unlikely to indirectly encourage murder. Gillam pointed out that the circumstances in both cases are very different (murder is widely condemned, abortion not; the moral status of a person is uncontroversial, that of a foetus is not, etc.). I think that there is reason to believe that the use of embryonic stem cells is more likely to encourage embryo destruction than the use of foetal tissue is likely to encourage abortion. This is because, by using embryonic stem cells, a researcher expresses support for the derivation of embryonic stem cells. We can safely assume she supports embryonic stem cell derivation, partly because she uses the stem cells for the purpose they were produced for.[29] (By contrast, we do not have any reason to assume that a researcher using foetal tissue supports abortion—the foetus was not aborted to

---

[28] McCormick et al., 'Distribution of Human Embryonic Stem Cell Lines', 108.

[29] Richard M. Doerflinger, 'The Ethics of Funding Embryonic Stem Cell Research: A Catholic Viewpoint', *Kennedy Institute of Ethics Journal*, 9 (1999), 137–50. Albert S. Moraczewski., 'May one Benefit from the Evil Deeds of Others?', *National Catholic Bioethics Quarterly*, 2 (2002), 43–7.

provide foetal tissue for research.) Expressing support for stem cell derivation, and thus embryo destruction, is likely to contribute to a wider tolerance of, or support for embryo destruction.

Expectably increasing the number of embryos destroyed

According to Singer, the fact that I buy the chicken instead of the tofu creates a demand for chicken. This will increase the supply of chicken in the supermarket, and thus the number of chickens slaughtered for consumption. Some may object to Singer's conclusion on the ground that the effect of an individual buying the chicken is too small to be perceived by the supermarket or the chicken industry. Hence it will not have any effect on the demand for chickens, and thus on the chicken supply. This would imply that you buying a chicken in the supermarket does not have any effect on the number of chickens slaughtered. Likewise, the effect of one researcher using embryonic stem cells on the demand for embryonic stem cells may be too small to be perceived by those producing embryonic stem cell lines. It may not have any impact on the embryonic stem cell supply, and, thus, on the number of embryos destroyed.

I believe, however, that, even if one's effect on the demand is small, or perhaps imperceptible, it may nevertheless be morally problematic. This is because an individual's small or even imperceptible effect *expectably*[30] makes a difference to the supply of chicken, and thus to the harm incurred on chickens.[31] An individual buying chicken in the supermarket *can* push the demand over the threshold required for the demand to be large enough to have an effect on the chicken supply (this is comparable to the voter who makes the difference between someone being elected or not[32]). Likewise, an individual researcher using embryonic stem cells *can* push the demand over the threshold that is required for it to be large enough to have an effect on the supply of embryonic stem

---

[30] The term 'expectably' is frequently used in economics and decision theory. I use 'expectably' here to refer to the mathematical concept of 'expected value'. According to that concept, if there is some (even a tiny) chance that the number of embryos killed will increase, and no chance that it will decrease, then the number of embryos expectably killed has increased.

[31] See also Kagan, 'Do I Make a Difference?'.

[32] For an analysis of the example of the voter's effect on elections, see Jonathan Glover and M. J. Scott-Taggart, 'It Makes No Difference Whether or Not I Do it', *Proceedings of the Aristotelian Society*, 49 (1975), 171–209.

cells, and thus, on the number of embryos destroyed. That she *expectably* encourages embryo destruction makes using embryonic stem cells in research presumptively wrong.

Even if a researcher, by using embryonic stem cells, does not push the demand over the threshold, she pushes it closer to it. By pushing the demand closer to the threshold, she contributes to the fact that someone will eventually push it *over* the threshold, which will result in more embryos being destroyed. This is especially problematic because the researcher *knows* that there are many other researchers who, just like her, push the demand closer to the threshold. She knows that she is a member of a group who together create a large enough demand for embryonic stem cells to result in more embryos destroyed. That her contribution to this demand, however minor, is problematic can be illustrated by Derek Parfit's famous case of the Harmless Torturers.[33] Parfit first introduces the Bad Old Days case where a thousand torturers have a thousand victims and where each torturer turns a switch on some kind of torture machine a thousand times. Each turn increases the victim's pain but in a way that is imperceptible to the victim. But when each torturer turns the switch a thousand times the victim suffers severe pain. Each torturer's action is clearly wrong. Parfit then introduces another case.

The Harmless Torturers: In the Bad Old Days, each torturer inflicted severe pain on one victim. Things have now changed. Each of the thousand torturers presses a button, thereby turning the switch once on each of the thousand instruments. The victims suffer the same severe pain. But none of the torturers makes any victim's pain perceptibly worse.[34]

Most would agree that in this case too, each torturer is acting wrongly (though they may disagree about why this is so). It is plausible that one reason why each torturer acts wrongly is that, even though each torturer's effect on the total harm is small or even imperceptible for the victim, it either brings the victim closer to the threshold needed to feel the pain, or pushes it over that threshold,[35] and this makes it

---

[33] Derek Parfit, *Reasons and Persons* (Oxford: Oxford University Press, 1984), 80.

[34] Parfit, *Reasons and Persons*, 80. Earlier, Glover had used the now famous '100 beans case' to make the same point. Glover and Scott-Taggart, 'It Makes No Difference'.

[35] According to Shelly Kagan, it is not possible that each individual torturer's act makes no difference to the pain experienced by the victim, yet enough such acts together do make

presumptively wrong—especially because the torturers know that their contribution will be topped up by other torturers.

The same is true for embryonic stem cell research. Suppose that an individual researcher using embryonic stem cells only has a slight impact on the demand that is required for there to be an effect on the total supply of embryonic stem cell lines. Even if the researcher does not push the demand over the threshold for such an effect to occur, using these embryonic stem cells is presumptively wrong because she thereby pushes the demand in the direction of the threshold. Like in *The Harmless Torturers*, a researcher using embryonic stem cells is not acting alone. There are many other researchers who also each have a slight effect on the demand. By using embryonic stem cells a researcher knowingly and intentionally contributes to this aggregate demand—a demand that *will* have an effect on the supply of embryonic stem cell lines, and thus on the numbers of embryos destroyed.

That the impact on the total number of embryos destroyed may be small (for example, because the supply of one extra embryonic stem cell line does only require the destruction of a few more embryos) should not make it less problematic. Even if an individual researcher, or a group of researchers, 'merely' using embryonic stem cells causes only one extra embryo's destruction of the many that are destroyed in any case, this should be considered presumptively wrong if the embryo has a significant moral status. This is especially clear if one accords a full moral status to the embryo. It would be presumptively wrong if I contributed to killing a person, even if a thousand other persons will be killed in any case. Even if I can only make a small difference to whether or not a person is killed, this difference matters. But even if one accords a somewhat lower moral status to the embryo, making this small difference matters and should be accounted for. If I object to the slaughtering of animals for meat, it is presumptively wrong to eat meat even if this results in only one animal extra slaughtered. Robertson's claim that encouraging embryonic stem cell research is only problematic if it results in a *significant* increase in the number of embryos destroyed is unconvincing.

But suppose that my argument to this point fails and that, by using embryonic stem cells, a researcher does *not* increase the number of

a difference. At least some torturers' acts must make a perceptible difference. Kagan, 'Do I Make a Difference?'.

embryos destroyed, not even expectably so. Suppose, for example, that those deriving embryonic stem cells only produce embryonic stem cell lines for their own research, and not for others' research, though they allow others to benefit from the stem cell lines they created for themselves. (So no new embryonic stem cell lines are created for others.) Would this be sufficient to show that merely using embryonic stem cells does not encourage wrongdoing in a way that makes it presumptively wrong?

Encouraging without increasing the number of embryos destroyed

There are many cases where an individual's encouragement of or participation in others' wrongdoing does not make a difference to the total incidence of the wrongdoing but where one nevertheless encourages or participates in wrongdoing in a way that is presumptively wrong.

Consider two cases where one participates in wrongdoing, without making a difference to the total incidence of the wrongdoing, but where it is intuitively clear that one's participation is presumptively wrong.

> *Platform*: you join four other people in pushing a big container on a platform in the hope that it will fall off the platform and will crush an innocent person. In fact, four men are needed to push the container off the platform.

> *Execution*: You are one of five soldiers who execute an innocent prisoner by simultaneously shooting him in the same spot. In fact, only one soldier's shot is needed to kill the prisoner.

Both cases are so-called overdetermination cases. The action of each man on the platform and each soldier is neither necessary nor sufficient for the wrongdoing to occur. Each individual's action nevertheless involves participating in the wrongdoing in a way that may be wrong. One plausible explanation for why this is so is that because together they cause the wrongdoing to occur. By being a part of such a group, one contributes to the bad effect, even though one's act was neither necessary nor sufficient for the wrongdoing to occur. Had each man acted differently, the victim would not have died.[36]

Likewise, one researcher using embryonic stem cells may be neither necessary nor sufficient to have an effect on the supply of embryonic

---

[36] Parfit, *Reasons and Persons*, 70–1.

stem cell lines. The researcher nevertheless encourages an increase in the supply of embryonic stem cells. That it is a case of encouragement of wrongdoing rather than direct participation in wrongdoing (like in Platform or Execution) is not morally important enough to prevent the contribution from being wrong itself. This can be shown by changing Platform as follows:

> *Platform**: Ten men promise a reward for those individuals who can push a big container on a platform in the hope that it will fall off the platform and will crush an innocent person. In fact, the encouragement of only five men is needed for the four men to push the container off the platform.

It is intuitively clear that all ten men who promise a reward encourage the wrongdoing even though each one's promise of a reward is neither necessary nor sufficient for the wrongdoing to occur. Each of them participates in the wrongdoing. Had each one of them acted differently, the wrongdoing would not have occurred.[37]

So it is plausible that one can encourage wrongdoing without making a difference to the total incidence of wrongdoing. It is thus plausible that by using embryonic stem cells, a researcher encourages embryo destruction, even if his research does not result in more embryos being destroyed than would otherwise be destroyed.

3.5. Cut-Off Dates do Not Avoid Encouragement

Some defenders of the use–derivation distinction acknowledge the problem that, by using embryonic stem cell lines, researchers in institutions and countries opposed to embryonic stem cell derivation always encourage embryo destruction. To avoid any encouragement of embryo destruction, Germany and the United States under Bush's governance decided to implement a more restrictive stem cell policy—though one that is still based on the use–derivation distinction.

Both countries introduced cut-off dates. In the US, federal funding would only be available for research using embryonic stem cells that had

---

[37] Parfit, *Reasons and Persons.*

been produced *before* 11 August 2001, when the new policy was announced. Bush explained that for the embryos used to produce these lines 'the life and death decision has already been made'. By restricting federal funding to embryonic stem cells produced before that cut-off date, federally funded scientists would be able

to explore the promise and potential of stem cell research without crossing a fundamental moral line, by providing taxpayer funding that would sanction or encourage further destruction of human embryos.[38]

Germany also introduced a cut-off date. Stem cell derivation is illegal in Germany, as the Embryo Protection Act of 1991 prohibits all embryo research that is not for the benefit of the embryo the research is conducted on. However, the German Stem Cell Law of 2002 tolerates the use of embryonic stem cells that were produced abroad before 1 January 2002. By introducing this cut-off date, Germany, like the US, intended to avoid any encouragement of the production of embryonic stem cells abroad. Thus, the idea was that Americans and Germans were permitted to enjoy the benefits of previous wrongdoing, without encouraging in any way the repetition of similar wrongdoing in the future.

But is it true that introducing a cut-off date avoids encouragement of embryo destruction all together? Again, I think the answer is negative.

First, by using embryonic stem cells produced before a cut-off date one is still likely to inspire and stimulate embryonic stem cell research in less restrictive countries or jurisdictions, where embryonic stem cell derivation *is* allowed. One may thereby, indirectly, encourage the destruction of embryos.[39] This concern was also the reason why some opponents of embryo destruction objected to Bush' embryonic stem cell policy.[40]

Second, a cut-off date is unlikely to stay in place. Once one accepts that a restricted number of cell lines can be used for research because of the great benefits of embryonic stem cell research, it becomes hard to resist not increasing this number when existing lines turn out to be insufficient

[38] White House, Office of the Press Secretary, 'Radio address by the President to the nation', Bush Ranch, Texas, 11 Aug. 2001, <www.whitehouse.gov/news/releases/2001/08/20010809-2.html>. For the eligibility criteria, see <http://stemcells.nih.gov/StaticResources/research/registry/pdfs/EligibilityCriteria.pdf>.

[39] Heidi Mertes and Guido Pennings, 'Stem Cell Research Policies: Who's Afraid of Complicity?', *Reproductive BioMedicine Online*, 19 (2009), 38–42.

[40] Doerflinger, 'Ethics of Funding'.

to achieve these benefits. This has already shown to be the case in Germany where the cut-off date was moved from 1 January 2002 to 1 May 2007. As pointed out by Louis Guenin, if it is known or anticipated that the government will periodically advance the cut-off date, then those producing embryonic stem cell lines will be induced to create new embryonic stem cell lines in expectation of the next advance.[41]

In the US, the cut-off date has been removed altogether. In March 2009, President Obama issued an executive order entitled 'Removing Barriers to Responsible Scientific Research Involving Human Stem Cells', which states that federal funding is no longer restricted to stem cell lines that were created before 11 August 2001. (However, the derivation of embryonic stem cells still cannot be funded, due to the Dickey-Wicker Amendment.). The executive order states that

Advances over the past decade in this promising scientific field have been encouraging, leading to broad agreement in the scientific community that the research should be supported by Federal funds.[42]

3.6. Conclusion

Before considering the arguments adduced in favour of the use–derivation distinction, I discussed a necessary assumption for this distinction to hold: that embryonic stem cells are not embryos or their moral equivalents. I argued that tetraploid complementation technology casts doubt on this assumption, at least if one accords a moral status to the embryo in virtue of its potential to develop into a person. Research involving tetraploid complementation suggests that embryonic stem cells, when provided with the right environment, can give rise to a person. This presents an interesting dilemma for those opposing the derivation of embryonic stem cells: if they continue to appeal to the potentiality argument, they also risk undermining the use of embryonic stem cells for research, and thus the use–derivation distinction. If they reject the potentiality argument, they must eschew restrictions on the

---

[41] Louis M. Guenin, 'A Failed Noncomplicity Scheme', *Stem Cells and Development*, 13 (2004), 456–9.

[42] White House, Office of the Press Secretary, *Executive Order: Removing Barriers to Responsible Scientific Research Involving Human Stem Cells*, section 1, 9 Mar. 2009. Available at <http://www.whitehouse.gov/the-press-office/removing-barriers-responsible-scientific-research-involving-human-stem-cells>.

derivation of embryonic stem cells or seek some other basis for them. Alternatively, they must find some way of distinguishing between the potential of embryonic stem cells and the potential of embryos. However, I have raised doubts on whether this can be done.

I then considered the most important argument adduced in defence of the use–derivation distinction: that, under the right conditions, using embryonic stem cells does not encourage embryo destruction. I argued that by using embryonic stem cells, a researcher always encourages embryo destruction in a way that makes it presumptively wrong. She does so by (i) increasing the number of embryos destroyed, (ii) expectably increasing the number of embryos destroyed, or (iii) being a necessary part of a group that is sufficient to expectably encourage embryo destruction. Finally, I argued that a cut-off date cannot rescue the argument that using embryonic stem cells does not encourage embryonic stem cell derivation. As has proven to be true, cut-off dates are unlikely to stay in place, and even if they did stay in place, researchers using embryonic stem cells would still indirectly encourage embryo destruction, by inspiring embryonic stem cell research in general. Thus, the main argument adduced in support of the use–derivation distinction faces serious problems. This suggests that, as long as no stronger arguments are presented, we should reject the use–derivation distinction as a correct ethical position.

4

Technical Solutions

4.1. Alternative Sources of Pluripotent Stem Cells

In Chapters 2 and 3, I focused on the first type of response that has been made to the Problem: the development of a middle-ground position intermediate between the dominant opposing views on the permissibility of embryonic stem cell research. The two middle-ground positions I discussed were the discarded–created distinction, which holds that it is permissible to use and derive stem cells from discarded embryos but not from research embryos, and the use–derivation distinction, which holds that it may be permissible to use but never to derive embryonic stem cells. I have shown that the arguments adduced in defence of these middle-ground positions are unconvincing or are inconsistently applied. Contrary to what their advocates sometimes claim, both middle-ground positions fail to offer a satisfying solution to the Problem.

However, there may be other solutions or ways to circumvent the Problem. Some have suggested that if embryonic stem cells, or their functional equivalents, could be created without destroying embryos, a good deal of the ethical controversy surrounding embryonic stem cell research would subside and the Problem would dissolve. This resulted in a growing trend to seek technical solutions to the problem of destroying embryos to obtain stem cells. In May 2005, the US President's Council on Bioethics published a white paper, *Alternative Sources of Pluripotent Stem Cells*, discussing four proposals to produce pluripotent stem cells without creating, harming, or destroying embryos.[1] One month after the publication of this white paper, Senator Roscoe Bartlett introduced Bill

---

[1] President's Council on Bioethics, *Alternative Sources of Pluripotent Stem Cells* (Washington, DC: President's Council on Bioethics, 2005).

HR3144, also known as the 'Respect for Life Pluripotent Stem Cell Act', proposing US$15 million a year for the development of 'embryonic stem cell alternatives that do not harm embryos'. The bill never became law but in September 2007 President Bush issued an executive order requiring that:

> The Secretary of Health and Human Services (Secretary) shall conduct and support research on the isolation, derivation, production, and testing of stem cells that are capable of producing all or almost all of the cell types of the developing body and may result in improved understanding of or treatments for diseases and other adverse health conditions, but are derived without creating a human embryo for research purposes or destroying, discarding, or subjecting to harm a human embryo or foetus.[2]

Shortly after the executive order was issued, the NIH announced that it would begin implementing it, exploring 'research on alternative sources of pluripotent stem cells, including specifically those techniques outlined in a 2005 white paper by the President's Council on Bioethics'.[3]

The case for supporting these proposals is obvious: their implementation holds the promise of advancing research with embryonic or other pluripotent stem cells, without becoming entangled in concerns regarding the moral status of the embryo. No extra embryos would be created, nor would any living embryo be subjected to dangerous manipulation or be destroyed. Would this not be the perfect solution to the Problem?

In this chapter, I examine the proposals for alternative sources of pluripotent stem cells discussed by the President's Council on Bioethics, as well as some proposals that have been advanced and pursued subsequently. I divide the proposed solutions in three groups: (1) techniques that use embryos, but avoid harming them, (2) techniques that use embryo-like entities that, arguably, are not embryos, and (3) techniques that involve the direct reprogramming of somatic cells.

---

[2] US Government, *Executive Order 13435: Expanding Approved Stem Cell Lines in Ethically Responsible Ways* (Federal Register, 22 June 2007), 34951–3, <http://edocket. access.gpo.gov/2007/pdf/07-3112.pdf>.

[3] Department of Health and Human Services and National Institutes of Health, *Plan for Implementation of Executive Order 13435: Expanding Approved Stem Cell Lines in Ethically Responsible Ways* (18 Sept. 2007), <http://stemcells.nih.gov/staticresources/policy/eo13435. pdf>.

4.2. Techniques that Avoid Harming Embryos

A first set of proposals involves techniques to derive embryonic stem cells without harming the embryo, either because the embryo is already dead, or because the embryo survives the derivation procedure.

Organismically dead embryos

In 2004, physicians Donald Landry and Howard Zucker proposed to use what they called 'organismically dead embryos' as a source of pluripotent stem cells.[4] These are IVF embryos that 'died spontaneously' during efforts to prepare them for transfer into the uterus. Landry and Zucker suggest that embryos should be considered dead when they have irreversibly lost 'the capacity for continued and integrated cellular division, growth, and differentiation'. This criterion, they say, is comparable to the standard definition of brain death, which 'marks the irreversible loss of the capacity for all ongoing and integrated organic functioning'.[5] Landry and Zucker claim that the strength of their proposal is that it is modelled after the ethical framework widely accepted for organ donation. In both cases, the individual (assuming the embryo is an individual) is what they call *organismically* but not thoroughly dead, which implies that some organs—or cells in the case of the embryo—may still be viable and, in most cases, can still be harvested for organ transplantation, or the generation of embryonic stem cell lines. The argument then is that, even if one accords a full moral status to the embryo, one can accept the derivation of stem cells from organismically dead embryos. After all, most people agree that full-grown human beings have full moral status but think that it may be permissible to harvest their organs for transplantation purposes once they are brain dead.

A first question to be asked when evaluating each proposed technique to derive pluripotent stem cells without harming embryos is whether it can really offer a scientifically and clinically useful alternative to embryonic stem cells from discarded embryos. Some have raised the concern that stem cells derived from organismically dead embryos would be of suboptimal quality as these embryos undergo developmental arrest

---

[4] Donald W. Landry and Howard A. Zucker, 'Embryonic Death and the Creation of Human Embryonic Stem Cells', *Journal of Clinical Investigation*, 114 (2004), 1184–6.
[5] Landry and Zucker, 'Embryonic Death', 1185.

(where the cells stop dividing and the embryo no longer grows) for a reason: often, embryos that underwent developmental arrest are genetically abnormal. This may influence their capacity to give rise to normal embryonic stem cell lines and may make them less suited for therapeutic use.[6] Several research teams have, however, succeeded in deriving embryonic stem cell lines with apparently normal chromosomes from arrested embryos. For example, George Daley's research team at Harvard showed that early arrested embryos are a poor source of embryonic stem cell lines, but that late arrested embryos (that is, embryos arrested in the blastocyst stage) have an efficiency of embryonic stem cell derivation similar to that of frozen embryos.[7] However, what these researchers emphasize is that, though organismically dead embryos may offer a valuable *extra* source of embryonic stem cells, they cannot be regarded as the *sole* source of embryonic stem cells. A Swiss research team that successfully derived stem cell lines from arrested embryos also concluded that

[a]s the destruction of viable developing embryos, even spare ones, raises serious ethical concerns, deriving hESC lines from arrested embryos may be an alternative approach to avoid embryo destruction. However, given the reduced derivation efficiency they should not be considered a unique and/or selective source of hESC lines.[8]

The reason given here for regarding organismically dead embryos as only a supplementary source of embryos is that the derivation procedure is not efficient. It should also be noted that, since stem cells from organismically dead IVF embryos would not typically be genetically identical to the patient, they would not offer an alternative to stem cells produced through SCNT.

Even setting aside these technical constraints, there is a further problem with the Landry-Zucker proposal: we can expect there to be wide disagreement on how to determine whether or not an embryo is

---

[6] Dusko Ilic et al., 'Effect of Karyotype on Successful Human Embryonic Stem Cell Derivation', *Stem Cells and Development*, 19 (2010), 39–46.

[7] Paul H. Lerou et al., 'Human Embryonic Stem Cell Derivation from Poor-Quality Embryos', *Nature Biotechnology*, 26 (2008), 212–14.

[8] Anis Feki et al., 'Derivation of the First Swiss Human Embryonic Stem Cell Line from a Single Blastomere of an Arrested Four-Cell-Stage Embryo', *Swiss Medical Weekly*, 138 (2009), 640–60. See, for a similar claim, Xin Zhang et al., 'Derivation of Human Embryonic Stem Cells from Developing and Arrested Embryos', *Stem Cells*, 24 (2006), 2669.

'organismically dead'. Some may argue that it might not even make sense to speak of 'death' when we are talking about very early embryos (in the same way that it would not make sense to talk about the death of a skin cell). The proposal is supposed to be attractive because it is based on a widely accepted model of organ procurement from brain-dead individuals. But the use of that model as the corner stone of the proposal is problematic. First, it is not clear how we can derive conclusions from the brain death of full-grown human beings to the death of embryos, as the latter are physiologically very different from the former. But second, and more importantly, what Landry and Zucker seem to ignore is that the concept of brain death is controversial itself. It is the subject of ongoing scientific and ethical debate. The same will be true for determining embryonic death. Landry and Zucker suggest ways to experiment with dying embryos in order to develop criteria for organismic death, thereby implicitly suggesting that the answer will be a purely scientific one. However, the definition of organismic death and how to determine it will also be the result of an ethical evaluation. The point of the concept of 'organismic death' (like the concept of 'brain death') is to mark a class of organisms that are in a state that is morally equivalent or similar to 'full' death. But there might be as much debate about when an embryo is in a state that is morally similar or equivalent to full death as there is about what moral status to accord to the embryo. For example, it might well be argued that organismically dead embryos are quite different, in moral terms, from fully dead embryos since they still contain viable cells with normal developmental potential (it is these cells that will be used to create an embryonic stem cell line).[9] If organismically dead embryos are not dead, or in a state that is sufficiently similar to death, then the Landry-Zucker proposal fails to offer a solution to the Problem.[10]

In response, it has been argued that organismically dead embryos, though possibly still living in some sense, nevertheless lack the 'intrinsic potential' for further development and that, therefore, nothing important is lost when they are destroyed to obtain stem cells. However, this argument is not entirely convincing. Some embryos declared organismically

[9] John R. Meyer, 'The Significance of Induced Pluripotent Stem Cells for Basic Research and Clinical Therapy', *Journal of Medical Ethics*, 3 (2008), 849–51.

[10] Søren Holm, ' "New Embryos": New Challenges for the Ethics of Stem Cell Research', *Cells Tissues Organs*, 187 (2008), 257–62.

dead may in fact just be poor-quality embryos, that is, embryos with genetic or morphological defects that are usually discarded if a couple undergoing IVF also produced normal embryos. Poor-quality embryos may, however, still have some 'intrinsic potential' to generate successful pregnancies. If a couple undergoing IVF produce only poor-quality embryos, they may be implanted anyway, and although the pregnancy rate is extremely low with such embryos, it is not zero.[11] This means that some embryos declared organismically dead may still be sufficiently alive to continue the path of further development. They might be more akin to severely disabled people than brain-dead people. Destroying such embryos for research, and depriving them of their chance, however minimal, to further develop should thus be unacceptable for those objecting to the destruction of 'ordinary' discarded embryos—the group to whom the Landry-Zucker proposal is primarily addressed.

Finally, there is another problem with the Landry-Zucker proposal, and that is the link between the use of organismically dead embryos and woman-friendly IVF. At first sight, the Landry-Zucker proposal seems to avoid this link as the stem cell researchers do not have to rely on a supply of surplus embryos donated for research; they can simply use embryos that died spontaneously in an effort to transfer them into the uterus of a woman undergoing IVF. However, the conclusion that this breaks any link with woman-friendly IVF is too quick. First, it should be noted that in countries that only allow embryo-friendly IVF, like Italy, the supply of organismically dead embryos would simply be too small to constitute a reliable source of embryonic stem cell line. This is because only embryos that happened to die in the brief period between creation and implant-ation could be used. If the Landry-Zucker method were only used in these countries, this would dramatically slow down progress in embry-onic stem cell research and thus would not really help to resolve the Problem. To satisfy scientific and clinical demand, it would be necessary to make use of the large number of embryos that die after cryopreserva-tion in woman-friendly IVF. Landry himself has confirmed this.[12] Thus,

---

[11] Personal communication with George Daley, director of the Harvard Stem Cell Institute.

[12] Svetlana Gavrilov, Virginia E. Papaioannou, and Donald W. Landry, 'Alternative Strategies for the Derivation of Human Embryonic Stem Cell Lines and the Role of Dead Embryos', *Current Stem Cell Research and Therapy*, 4 (2009), 81–6.

stem cell derivation of organismically dead embryos is only a realistic solution to the Problem where there is woman-friendly IVF.

As Giuseppe Testa has pointed out, it is rather astonishing that defenders of the proposal ignore this link with woman-friendly IVF. Testa writes that

what this proposal tries to do is to re-establish in this very setting [of IVF] the narrative of the natural life cycle. After we have set the whole process [of IVF] in motion, we can, and in fact we should, leave a neutral space to watch unfolding the natural life of in vitro embryos. We should import the categories of natural life and natural death, shedding the normativity and intentionality that we have followed so far in order to watch the IVF embryos 'die on their own', as if watching artificially generated embryos die 'naturally' could claim back the naturalness for the whole process.[13]

Testa is right. The proposal seems to ignore the strong link with woman-friendly IVF, which is not a spontaneous or natural process. This is especially astonishing because the embryos' 'spontaneous' death can often be attributed at least in part to the freezing process, a necessary aspect of woman-friendly IVF (but not of embryo-friendly IVF). If the embryo has a significant moral status, one could argue that it should not have been subjected to such risks in the first place. This implies that one should also not encourage subjecting embryos to such risks. Moreover, as I argued in section 3.3, by routinely benefiting from woman-friendly IVF, a researcher may indirectly encourage embryo destruction. The fact that the embryos are organismically dead (if they are) does not avoid this problem. By routinely using these embryos in research, a researcher condones woman-friendly IVF, thereby encouraging it. It seems inconsistent to care so much about not destroying embryos for research while accepting the significant risks that woman-friendly IVF imposes on embryos.

For those who really oppose harming embryos, whether in the context of research or IVF, the Landry-Zucker proposal cannot offer a satisfactory solution to the Problem. It involves the risk of destroying still living embryos, and it indirectly encourages woman-friendly IVF, and thus the harm to embryos that comes along with that.

---

[13] Guiseppe Testa, 'Stem Cells through Stem Beliefs: The Co-production of Biotechnological Pluralism', *Science as Culture*, 17 (2008), 440.

Embryo biopsy

Another proposal to obtain embryonic stem cells without *harming* embryos involves the application of embryo biopsy. The idea here is that scientists could produce an embryonic stem cell line from one cell—a blastomere—biopsied from an eight-cell stage embryo without impeding that embryo's development. The technique to biopsy one cell from an early embryo without compromising the embryo's developmental potential has been routine for more than three decades in the context of fertility treatments. When a couple wishes to prevent transferring a particular genetic disease to their child, they can make use of IVF combined with preimplantation genetic diagnosis (PGD). In PGD, one cell of each (good-quality) embryo created via IVF is biopsied and subsequently tested for that particular genetic disease. Only embryos that turn out not to be carriers of the gene associated with the disease will be transferred to the uterus.

If embryo biopsy was performed in the context of embryonic stem cell research, the biopsied cells would not be used for genetic testing; they would instead be used to produce an embryonic stem cell line. This was shown to be technically feasible in 2006, when Advanced Cell Technology first reported the successful generation of human embryonic stem cell lines from cells biopsied from early-stage embryos.[14] Since the biopsied cells are blastomeres, I refer to this proposed alternative as 'blastomere biopsy'.

Does blastomere biopsy offer a solution to the Problem?

A major concern is that some early-stage blastomeres may not be pluripotent but totipotent. If a blastomere is totipotent then, once removed from an embryo, it could be regarded as a new embryo in its own right since it has the capacity to develop into a person. Using a totipotent blastomere to produce an embryonic stem cell line would thus involve embryo destruction.[15] To avoid this problem, ethicist Matthew Liao proposed a variant of blastomere biopsy, which he called the 'blastocyst transfer method' (BTM).[16] This procedure also involves

---

[14] Irina Klimanskaya et al., 'Human Embryonic Stem Cell Lines Derived from Single Blastomeres', *Nature*, 444 (2006), 481–5.

[15] John R. Meyer, 'Human Embryonic Stem Cells and Respect for Life', *Journal of Medical Ethics*, 26 (2000), 166–70.

[16] Matthew S. Liao, 'Rescuing Human Embryonic Stem Cell Research: The Blastocyst Transfer Method', *American Journal of Bioethics*, 5 (2005), 8–16.

embryo biopsy but at a later stage of the embryo's development—at the blastocyst stage. The idea is that the biopsied cells from the blastocyst are definitely no longer totipotent but merely pluripotent, and thus cannot be regarded as embryos in their own right.

Aside from any technical hurdles with BTM, I believe that it too fails to circumvent the ethical issues raised by embryonic stem cell research. First, the technique could only be developed and perfected through experiments that involve destroying or exposing at least some embryos to significant risks of harm. Liao takes this concern seriously but suggests that it can be met by organizing BTM experiments in such a way that no human embryos would need to be harmed.[17] He proposes that, initially, BTM research should only be done on animals. Only when the technique is considered safe in animals should we proceed to experiments with human embryos. At the start of these 'human trials', BTM should only be applied 'to embryos that have serious diseases and that could directly benefit from stem cell therapy'.[18] With this Liao means that the person the embryo gives rise to will be able to benefit from stem cell therapy. She will have her own, genetically identical embryonic stem cell line that can be used to treat her disease. Liao proposes that, to identify embryos with a serious disease, we could first look at family history and then apply PGD to confirm the diagnosis. The idea is that, although BTM imposes some risk on the embryo, this risk is outweighed by the significant gains for the person the embryo will give rise to.

However, a first problem with this approach is that it requires PGD. Those who believe that an embryo is a person are typically opposed to PGD, since it imposes a serious risk on the embryo (it might not survive the procedure). Carson Strong pointed out another problem with BTM. One may wonder which parents will select an embryo that is known to be a carrier of a serious genetic disease for transfer to the uterus, even if there is a therapy available to treat the disease?[19] Although those who accord a significant moral status to the embryo would perhaps want such embryos to be transferred to the uterus (as having a disease does not affect moral status), a couple undergoing

[17] Liao, 'Rescuing Human Embryonic Stem Cell Research', 14.

[18] Liao, 'Rescuing Human Embryonic Stem Cell Research', 14.

[19] Carson Strong, 'Obtaining Stem Cells: Moving from Scylla toward Charybdis', *American Journal of Bioethics*, 5 (2005), 21–3.

IVF are unlikely to want that. If their embryos run a high risk of being carriers of a serious genetic disease, the couple will typically make use of PGD in order to select the embryo that is *not* a carrier. If all embryos are carriers, they may prefer to undergo another IVF cycle to selecting an embryo with a genetic predisposition for a serious disease. A third problem is that embryonic stem cell therapy is still at the experimental stage and the chances that embryonic stem cell treatments will be developed by the time the individual needs treatment are low. Finally, BTM faces another problem. Even when further developed, BTM will remain an invasive technique and will expose the embryo to harm that reduces its viability. (The same is true for blastomere biopsy.) Liao writes that, for BTM to be permissible, its safety should be at the level of risk that is comparable to that of IVF and PGD.[20] However, as mentioned earlier, the reason why many who accord a significant moral status to the embryo object to IVF and PGD is precisely that it imposes extra risks on the embryos. If the embryo has a significant moral status, imposing such risks should indeed be considered unacceptable.[21] Note that the fact that embryo biopsy, performed at any stage of the embryo's development, exposes the embryo to risks it would otherwise not be exposed to, is also the reason why in the US, blastomere biopsy falls under the Dickey-Wicker Amendment and is thus not federally funded. It would knowingly subject embryos to significant risk of injury or death.

Neither blastomere biopsy nor BTM offer a satisfactory solution to the Problem. The biopsied blastomeres may be totipotent, and thus embryos themselves, and both blastomere biopsy and BTM expose embryos to a risk they would otherwise not be exposed to, without there being a benefit for the embryo that could outweigh that risk.

4.3. Techniques that Use Embryo-Like Entities

Another set of proposals involves the creation of biological artefacts as a source of pluripotent stem cells: artificially created entities that sufficiently resemble embryos to use as a source of pluripotent stem cells, but that, arguably, are not embryos so that destroying them is ethically

---

[20] Liao, 'Rescuing Human Embryonic Stem Cell Research', 12.
[21] See, also, Holm, ' "New Embryos": New Challenges'.

unproblematic. Whilst one still destroys something, one does not destroy an *embryo*.

Altered Nuclear Transfer

It was William Hurlbut, a physician and ethicist from Stanford University, who first proposed the creation of such biological artefacts as a solution to the Problem. He advocated a method that resembles SCNT but that involves the genetic alteration of the nucleus of the donor cell so that, when introduced into an enucleated egg, the resulting entity starts dividing but will not develop into an embryo. He called the method 'altered nuclear transfer' (ANT). Hurlbut explained that

> The resulting cells would have no inherent principle of unity, no coherent drive in the direction of the mature human form, and no claim on the moral status due to a developing human life. Rather, such a partial disorganized organic potential would more rightly be designated a 'biological artifact'—a human creation for human ends.[22]

The idea is that, since an entity resulting from ANT (for brevity's sake, I will refer to such an entity as an ANTity) is not an embryo, it is ethically unproblematic to destroy it in order to obtain pluripotent stem cells. Moreover, ANTity-derived stem cells would be 'customized' stem cells—they would be genetically identical to the donor of the somatic cell, for example, the patient. Thus, it seems like ANT could offer an embryo-friendly alternative to SCNT.

Hurlbut stresses that there are numerous ways in which ANTities could be created. The technique he suggests involves turning off the Cdx2 gene, which is required for the development of the trophectoderm, and thus the placenta. In mice, when Cdx2 is not expressed there is only a partial and disorganized developmental process. The resulting ANTity cannot implant in the uterus. However, an inner cell mass is formed from which functional embryonic stem cells can be harvested. In 2006, Alexander Meissner and Rudolf Jaenisch from the Whitehead Institute in Cambridge, Massachusetts, provided proof of principle for ANT-Cdx2

---

[22] William B. Hurlbut, 'Altered Nuclear Transfer as a Morally Acceptable Means for the Procurement of Human Embryonic Stem Cells', *Perspectives in Biology and Medicine*, 48 (2005), 211–28.

in the mouse.[23] The mouse ANTities were unable to implant in the uterus and the scientists succeeded in deriving pluripotent stem cells from the ANTities.

Can ANT offer a scientifically and clinically useful alternative to deriving embryonic stem cells from embryos? Scientists have pointed out that embryonic stem cells carrying a mutation in Cdx2 will be restricted in their developmental capacity in ways that may limit their usefulness in research and clinical applications.[24] The manipulation needed to control Cdx2 expression also makes the technique highly complicated and labour-intensive. The technique is based on SCNT, which is complicated in itself. But ANT requires additional manipulations, which further complicates the logistics of production and safety assessment of the cells.

But suppose ANT was an efficient way to produce embryonic stem cell lines, would it avoid the ethical issues? Again, I think the answer is negative.

Meissner and Jaenisch emphasize that mouse ANTities are not *human* ANTities, and that in order to know whether this technique could be used to generate *human* pluripotent stem cells further experiments must be done with primate and human cells. But these experiments would involve embryo destruction, and would thus be problematic if embryos have a significant moral status. Thus a first problem is that the development of ANT (just like the development of BTM) requires experiments in which embryos are destroyed.[25]

But the question that has been at the heart of the ethical debate is whether it is plausible to assume that an ANTity is not an embryo, or its moral equivalent. According to Hurlbut, an advantage of his proposal is that it

shifts the ethical debate from the question of *when* a normal embryo is a human being with moral worth, to the more fundamental question of *what* component parts and organized structure constitute the minimal criteria for considering an entity a human organism.[26]

---

[23] Alexander Meissner and Rudolph Jaenisch, 'Generation of Nuclear Transfer-Derived Pluripotent ES Cells from Cloned Cdx2-Deficient Blastocysts', *Nature*, 439 (2006), 212–15.

[24] Douglas A. Melton, George Q. Daley, and Charles G. Jennings, 'Altered Nuclear Transfer in Stem-Cell Research: A Flawed Proposal', *New England Journal of Medicine*, 351 (2004), 2791–2.

[25] See also Roberto Colombo, 'Altered Nuclear Transfer', *Communio*, 31 (2004), 645–8.

[26] William B. Hurlbut, 'Altered Nuclear Transfer as a Morally Acceptable Means for the Procurement of Human Embryonic Stem Cells', paper presented to the President's Council

It is, however, doubtful whether the last question will be more easily answered than the former, as there is no consensus on the definition of an embryo, or a human organism for that matter. Again, this is not only a matter of scientific facts, but also of ethical evaluation. Hurlbut emphasizes that a crucial feature of his proposal is that the genetic alteration is done right from the start, that is, before an embryo comes into being. But although the alteration is done at the start, the Cdx2 gene is not expressed until the morula stage. As a result, its knock-down effect does not take place until then. This suggests that the ANTity is in fact a normal embryo that happens to be programmed for an early death; indeed, some have referred to it as 'a normal but short lived embryo', or 'a disabled embryo'.[27] This is plausible. A newborn baby that will only live for five days is still a baby, even if it was programmed from the start that it would only live for five days. Several stem cell scientists seem to agree with this observation. For example, Meissner and Jaenisch point out that 'because the Cdx2-deficient embryo is not obviously abnormal before the onset of Cdx2 expression, this approach may not solve the ethical dilemma'. Douglas Melton, George Daley, and Charles Jennings also believe that ANTities are in fact embryos that develop normally until CDX2 function is required, at which point they die.[28]

The fact that an ANTity would be developing normally until the expression of Cdx2 raises another problem. If it is acceptable to produce an ANTity that develops normally for four days before becoming what Hurlbut calls 'disorganized growth', it should also be acceptable to develop an ANTity that develops much longer, say ten weeks, before it becomes disorganized growth. My hunch is, however, that creating ten-week-old ANTities as a source of stem cells (or organs) would not be considered an acceptable alternative to ordinary embryonic stem cell or foetal tissue research. If embryos, just like ten-week old foetuses, have a significant moral status, then the destruction of say three-day old ANTities should be considered unacceptable too.

---

on Bioethics on 3 Dec. 2004, <http://bioethics.georgetown.edu/pcbe/background/hurlbut.html>.

[27] Colombo, 'Altered Nuclear Transfer'. William J. Burke et al., 'Stemming the Tide of Cloning', *First Things*, 158 (2005), 7. Hans Werner Denker, 'Induced Pluripotent Stem Cells: How to Deal with the Developmental Potential', *Reproductive BioMedicine Online*, 19 (2009), 34–7.

[28] Melton et al., 'Altered Nuclear Transfer in Stem-Cell Research'.

To overcome the concerns raised by the apparent normal but short embryonic development of Cdx2-ANTities, a group of thirty-five ethicists and scientists proposed a variation of ANT, which they named 'oocyte assisted reprogramming' (OAR). This technique would involve the application of ANT, but in such a way that the genetic alteration would take effect *immediately*.[29] This would be done by overexpression of the transcription factor Nanog both in the enucleated oocyte and in the somatic cell prior to transfer of its nucleus. Nanog is known to play a central role in maintaining pluripotency in mouse embryonic stem cells. The idea behind this proposal is that an ANTity resulting from OAR would *immediately* be pluripotent. At no point would an embryo be formed. According to the authors, the characteristics of the resulting entity would 'from the beginning be clearly and unambiguously distinct from, and incompatible with, those of an embryo'.[30]

This proposal has been criticized both for being scientifically unrealistic and for failing to escape the ethical issues. It has been argued that the proposal is based on a flawed understanding of stem cell biology because it is unlikely that Nanog is in itself able to transform a newly cloned embryo into a pluripotent cell.[31] This is because the oocyte is an extremely powerful reprogramming cell itself. It could well be the case that factors in the oocyte cytoplasm may overwhelm the presence of Nanog and steer development on a normal course to further embryonic development.

But even if the proposal were scientifically realistic, it would not avoid the issue of embryo destruction. ANTities with an overexpressed Nanog gene could, just like ANTities in which Cdx2 has been suppressed, be regarded as disabled embryos. In the normal zygote, Nanog prevents the cells from differentiating past a certain stage of development. It keeps pluripotent cells pluripotent. Overexpressing Nanog in an ANTity could easily be interpreted as producing a disabled embryo incapable of developing further.[32]

---

[29] Hadley Arkes, et al., 'Production of Pluripotent Stem Cells by Oocyte-Assisted Reprogramming: Joint Statement with Signatories', *National Catholic Bioethics Quarterly*, 5 (2005), 579–83.

[30] Arkes et al., 'Production of Pluripotent Stem Cells', 579.

[31] W. Malcolm Byrnes, 'The Flawed Scientific Basis of the Altered Nuclear Transfer-Oocyte Assisted Reprogramming (ANT-OAR) Proposal', *Stem Cell Review*, 1 (2007), 63.

[32] David L. Schindler, 'A Response to the Joint Statement, "Production of Pluripotent Stem Cells by Oocyte Assisted Reprogramming"', *Communio*, 32 (Summer 2005).

That the alterations in ANTities could be reversed (both the over-expression of Nanog and the suppression of Cdx2) only seems to confirm that ANTities are in fact disabled embryos.[33] The reversibility of the alterations also raises the question whether, if the embryo has a significant moral status, we should not rather rescue it by activating or deactivating the altered gene, instead of destroying it in research.

ANTities are unlikely to offer a scientifically and clinically useful alternative to embryonic stem cells from SCNT embryos, but even if they did, the problem of embryo destruction would not be solved. The development of ANT requires research that involves embryo destruction, and it is plausible to think of ANTities—whether those in which Cdx2 is suppressed or Nanog is overexpressed—as normal but short-lived embryos. Destroying them would thus be unacceptable if the embryo has a significant moral status.

Parthenogenesis

Parthenogenesis is a form of asexual reproduction in which oocytes can develop into embryos without being fertilized by sperm. The oocytes form so-called 'virgin-birth embryos'. Parthenogenesis occurs naturally in some invertebrate animal species (for example, in some bees and wasps, and in ants and flies) and in some vertebrates (for example, in snakes, lizards, and fish). It is not known to occur naturally in mammals. However, with the right chemicals, mammalian parthenotes, including *human* parthenotes, can be created *in vitro*. Because mammalian parthenotes contain only egg-derived DNA, they lack the genetic imprinting required for developing to term. Mammalian parthenotes created *in vitro* can undergo several cycles of cell division, but they are not viable embryos. Some mammalian parthenotes can develop through gastrulation (when the primitive streak is formed in the place where the backbone will later develop, around week two after conception) and early stages of organogenesis when transferred to a uterus.[34]

Human parthenotes never develop past a few days. This suggests, according to some, that parthenotes are not really embryos and could thus be used as an ethically unproblematic source of embryonic

[33] Melton et al., 'Altered Nuclear Transfer in Stem-Cell Research'.
[34] Jose B. Cibelli, Kerrianne Cunniff, and Kent E. Vrana, 'Embryonic Stem Cells from Parthenotes', *Methods in Enzymology*, 418 (2006), 117–35.

stem cells.[35] Unlike with organismically dead embryos and ANTities, there is no method to 'rescue' parthenotes. Even when supplied with trophoblast cells, parthenotes stop developing and perish. Another advantage of parthenogenetic stem cells over 'ordinary' embryonic stem cells is that parthenote-derived embryonic stem cells are a closer match to the oocyte donor than embryonic stem cells derived from discarded embryos would be.

Several research teams have derived embryonic stem cells from human parthenotes created *in vitro*.[36] However, it remains to be seen how genetically stable and safe parthenote-derived embryonic stem cells are.[37] It is as yet not clear whether the fact that parthenotes originate from maternal cells only will limit their use in research and potential clinical applications.[38]

But even if parthenotes could be used as an alternative source of pluripotent stem cells, the question remains whether their use would avoid the ethical issues raised by ordinary embryonic stem cell research. The moral status of the parthenote is controversial.

Donald Bruce of the Church of Scotland, stated that

the moral status of parthenogenetic creations is not clear. If they are not viable because certain crucial factors in their development do not follow the pattern of normal sperm plus egg embryos, are these defective human embryos, or are they not real embryos at all?[39]

Jacques Suaudau, from the Pontifical Academy for Life, wrote that

In their view this parthenote, incapable of developing beyond the blastocyst stage, with no future potential, should be considered potentially dead, an apparent

---

[35] T. A. L. Brevini and F. Gandolfi, 'Parthenotes as a Source of Embryonic Stem Cells', *Cell Proliferation*, 41 (2008), 20–30.

[36] Ge Lin, et al., 'A Highly Homozygous and Parthenogenetic Human Embryonic Stem Cell Line Derived from a One-Pronuclear Oocyte Following in vitro Fertilization Procedure', *Cell Research*, 17 (2007), 999–1007. Qingyun Mai, et al., 'Derivation of Human Embryonic Stem Cell Lines from Parthenogenetic Blastocysts', *Cell Research*, 17 (2007), 1008–19. Elena S. Revazova et al., 'HLA Homozygous Stem Cell Lines Derived from Human Parthenogenetic Blastocysts: Cloning Stem Cells', *Cloning Stem Cells*, 9 (2007), 432–49. Brevini and Gandolfi, 'Parthenotes'.

[37] F. Pellestor, B. Andreo, T. Anahory, and S. Hamamah, 'The Occurrence of Aneuploidy in Human: Lessons from the Cytogenetic Studies of Human Oocytes', *European Journal of Medical Genetics*, 49 (2006), 103–16. Cibelli et al., 'Embryonic Stem Cells from Parthenotes'.

[38] Brevini and Gandolfi, 'Parthenotes'.

[39] Donald Bruce, 'Parthenogenetic Embryos don't Solve Embryo Ethical Problems', press release, Feb. 2002, <http://archive.srtp.org.uk/clonin79.htm>.

organism breaking down, and treated as such. This opinion seems questionable however, as these activated human oocytes behave exactly like normal embryos until their epigenetic imbalance curbs their development and stops them implanting in utero.[40]

According to Guido de Wert and Christine Mummery, a parthenote should be regarded as an embryo, because it undergoes the first cell divisions normally, though a non-viable one.[41]

Parthenotes could be a valuable additional source of embryonic stem cells. Their role in regenerative medicine still has to be determined. However, the moral status of parthenotes is controversial. They too could plausibly be regarded as disabled embryos.

4.4. Direct Reprogramming of Somatic Cells

None of the proposals discussed to derive embryonic stem cells without harming embryos seems to offer a true ethical alternative to ordinary embryonic stem cell research. Nevertheless, research into some of the proposed techniques continues as they are believed to offer valuable *additional* sources of embryonic stem cells. There is, however, one alternative way of producing pluripotent stem cells that I have not yet mentioned: the direct reprogramming of somatic cells to a pluripotent state. Many believe that this offers the long-sought solution to the Problem.

Induced pluripotent stem cells

In November 2007, two separate research teams—one led by Shinya Yamanaka from Kyoto University and one led by James Thomson from the University of Wisconsin—announced that they had reprogrammed human adult fibroblasts (skin cells) back to an embryonic stem cell-like state, but without using cloning technology. Cloning technology enables the *indirect* reprogramming of somatic cells. Indirect because, in order to derive pluripotent cells, first an embryo needs to

---

[40] J. Suaudeau, 'From Embryonic Stem Cells to iPS: An Ethical Perspective'. *Cell Proliferation*, 44 (2011), 70–84.

[41] Guido de Wert and Christine Mummery, 'Human Embryonic Stem Cells: Research, Ethics and Policy', *Human Reproduction*, 18 (2003), 672–82.

be created from the somatic cell. Yamanaka and Thomson had *directly* reprogrammed the skin cells, without creating an embryo as an intermediate step. Yamanaka's group reported in the journal *Cell* that it had produced 'human induced pluripotent stem cells' (iPSCs) using the same method they had previously shown to work in mice.[42] The scientists generated the iPSCs via genetic manipulation. Using retroviruses, they inserted four transcription factors into the genome of human fibroblasts.[43] This induced overexpression of four genes known to be actively expressed in embryonic stem cells. The resulting cells showed the essential characteristics of embryonic stem cells: they were pluripotent and when placed in culture they differentiated into several types of specialized body cells, including cardiac muscle cells and neurons. On the same day Yamanaka's paper was published, Thomson's research team reported similar results in the journal *Science*.[44] Soon afterwards, researchers from various other research institutions replicated and improved upon the results, and provided proof of principle for the potential use of iPSCs in therapy. For example, Jaenisch's research group showed that symptoms of sickle cell anaemia can be reduced with iPSCs in the mouse.[45] Just like SCNT, the iPSC technique could allow the generation of customized pluripotent stem cells, for example, pluripotent stem cells genetically identical to a patient. However, unlike SCNT, the iPSC technique does not rely on a supply of donor oocytes or the creation and destruction of embryos.

Finally, a solution to the problem?

It should then come as no surprise that many have welcomed the iPSC technique as the long-sought solution to the ethical issues raised by embryonic stem cell research. The President's Council on Bioethics,

---

[42] Kazutoshi Takahashi and Shinya Yamanaka, 'Induction of Pluripotent Stem Cells from Mouse Embryonic and Adult Fibroblast Cultures by Defined Factors', *Cell*, 126 (2006), 663–76. Kazutoshi Takahashi et al., 'Induction of Pluripotent Stem Cells from Adult Human Fibroblasts by Defined Factors', *Cell*, 131 (2007), 861–72.

[43] The four transcription factors were Oct3/4, Sox2, c-Myc, and Klf4.

[44] They used different transcription factors (OCT4, SOX2, NANOG, and LIN28) to reprogramme somatic cell nuclei to an undifferentiated state. Junying Yu et al. 'Induced Pluripotent Stem Cell Lines Derived from Human Somatic Cells', *Science*, 318 (2007), 1917–20.

[45] Jacob Hanna et al., 'Treatment of Sickle Cell Anemia Mouse Model with iPS Cells Generated from Autologous Skin', *Science*, 318 (2007), 1920–3.

which was mostly opposed to embryonic stem cell research, called direct reprogramming 'ethically unproblematic'.[46] Charles Krauthammer, one of the Council's members, wrote about iPSC research that 'the embryonic stem cell debate is over' now that there is 'an ethically neutral way to produce stem cells'.[47] Archbishop Rino Fisichella, then president of the Pontifical Academy for Life, said that 'with the development of iPS cells, the ethical debate that has raged in public opinion, parliaments and the scientific community can now be considered closed'.[48] Opponents of embryonic stem cell research have not been alone in welcoming iPSC research as an ethical alternative for obtaining pluripotent stem cells; those who accept embryonic stem cell research have also expressed their relief and contentment. Developmental neurobiologists Mahendra Rao and Maureen Condic write that

> Despite remaining technical hurdles, direct reprogramming represents an exceptionally promising and ethically uncompromised method for generating patient-specific stem cells for both research and therapeutic purposes.[49]

But is it true that the iPSC technique marks the end of the embryonic stem cell debate? By now you will be unsurprised to hear that, in what follows, I argue it is not.

iPSCs cannot replace embryonic stem cells

Those who have claimed that the embryonic stem cell debate is over assume, sometimes implicitly, that iPSC research can replace embryonic stem cell research. For example, when stating that the embryonic stem cell debate is over, Krauthammer seemed convinced that '[s]cientific reasons alone will now incline even the most willful researchers to leave the human embryo alone'.[50] However, it is becoming increasingly clear that iPSC research will not be able to *replace*

---

[46] President's Council on Bioethics, *Alternative Sources*, 59.

[47] Charles Krauthammer, 'Stem Cell Vindication for Bush', *Washington Post*, 30 Nov. 2007, A23, <http://www.washingtonpost.com/wp-dyn/content/article/2007/11/29/AR2007112901878.html>.

[48] Cited in 'Science: Adult Stem Cells More Promising than Embryonic', *Christian Telegraph*, accessed Feb. 2014, <www.christiantelegraph.com/issue7717.html>.

[49] Mahendra Rao and Maureen L. Condic, 'Alternative Sources of Pluripotent Stem Cells', *Stem Cells and Development*, 17 (2008), 4.

[50] Krauthammer, 'Stem Cell Vindication for Bush'.

embryonic stem cell research, at least not in the short- or medium-term future.[51]

One reason is that iPSC research is still in the very early stages. Research with iPSCs requires constant comparisons with embryonic stem cell research, which is still considered the gold standard.[52] For example, recent research has highlighted the need to improve the differentiation potency of iPSCs and this requires comparisons with embryonic stem cells.[53] Stem cell scientist Kevin Eggan writes that, to validate and improve iPSCs, scientists will 'need to make huge [numbers] of these cells from many different people and compare them in a battery of tests with human ES cells'.[54] The fact that most papers on iPSC research cite embryonic stem cell research also confirms the necessity of these comparisons.[55]

Juan Carlos Belmonte, from the Center of Regenerative Medicine in Barcelona, writes that

[w]e should definitely continue to work on ES cells, as they are the 'gold standard' against which we compare iPS cells. ES cells are needed to understand the basic mechanism of pluripotency and self-renewal. As such, it is out of the question to even suggest phasing them out. We will be lost without them.[56]

In a similar vein, Konrad Hochedlinger, stem cell scientist at Harvard University, writes that

once we have a better understanding of what iPS cells can do and what they cannot do—if anything—it will be worthwhile to revisit the question

---

[51] Kristina Hug and Göran Hermerén, 'Do we Still Need Human Embryonic Stem Cells for Stem Cell-Based Therapies? Epistemic and Ethical Aspects', *Stem Cell Reviews and Reports*, 7 (2011), 761–74.

[52] George Q. Daley et al., 'Broader Implications of Defining Standards for the Pluripotency of iPSCs', *Cell Stem Cell*, 4 (2009), 200–20. Juan Carlos Izpisúa Belmonte et al., 'Induced Pluripotent Stem Cells and Reprogramming: Seeing the Science through the Hype', *Nature Review Genetics*, 10 (2009), 878–83. Monya Baker, 'iPS Cells: Potent Stuff', *Nature Methods* 7 (2010), 17–19.

[53] Bao-Yang Hu et al., 'Neural Differentiation of Human Induced Pluripotent Stem Cells Follows Developmental Principles But with Variable Potency', *Proceedings of the National Academy of Sciences USA*, 107 (2010), 4335–40.

[54] Cited in Constance Holden and Gretchen Vogel, 'A Seismic Shift for Stem Cell Research', *Science*, 319 (2008), 560–3.

[55] Christopher Thomas Scott et al., 'Democracy Derived? New Trajectories in Pluripotent Stem Cell Research', *Cell*, 145 (2011), 820–6.

[56] Belmonte et al., 'Induced Pluripotent Stem Cells and Reprogramming'.

of whether ES cells have become obsolete. At the moment, this is clearly not the case.

A second reason why iPSC research is unlikely to replace embryonic stem cell research is that iPSCs and embryonic stem cells seem to be different in important ways.[57] Thus, it may turn out that embryonic stem cell research is most useful for some purposes, and iPSC research is most useful for others. For example, according to George Daley, embryonic stem cells derived from SCNT embryos will allow us to study early human development, which is not possible through iPSC research.[58] Scientific experiments also suggest that for some diseases embryonic stem cells are better for modelling the genetic basis, whereas iPSCs are better for modelling the actual expression of the disease.[59]

In a review article 'The Promise of Induced Pluripotent Stem Cells in Research and Therapy', Daisy Robinton and George Daley write:

> The differences between iPS cells and ES cells, as well as those among iPS cells, clearly affect the utility of these cells in research, disease modelling and therapeutics ... The differences do not diminish the potential of iPS cells, given that iPS cells have considerable advantages over ES cells. Rather than replacing ES cells with iPS cells, it is becoming clear that these two cell types complement one another.[60]

Many questions about the properties and the potential of embryonic stem cells and iPSCs are still open, but most scientists agree that at this time there is no reason to believe that iPSC research makes embryonic stem cell research obsolete.[61] This is the first reason why the embryonic stem cell debate is not over yet. The second reason, which I will discuss in the next section, is directly related to the first.

---

[57] Mark H. Chin et al., 'Induced Pluripotent Stem Cells and Embryonic Stem Cells are Distinguished by Gene Expression Signatures', *Cell Stem Cell*, 5 (2009), 111–23. Kathrin Plath and William E. Lowry, 'Progress in Understanding Reprogramming to the Induced Pluripotent State', *Nature Review Genetics*, 12 (2011), 253–65.

[58] Cited in Holden and Vogel, 'Seismic Shift'.

[59] Achia Urbach et al., 'Differential Modeling of Fragile X Syndrome by Human Embryonic Stem Cells and Induced Pluripotent Stem Cells', *Cell Stem Cell*, 6 (2010), 407–11.

[60] Daisy A. Robinton and George Q. Daley, 'The Promise of Induced Pluripotent Stem Cells in Research and Therapy', *Nature* 481 (2012), 300.

[61] Holden and Vogel, 'Seismic Shift'. Belmonte et al., 'Induced Pluripotent Stem Cells and Reprogramming'. Hug and Hermerén, 'Still Need Human Embryonic Stem Cells'.

iPSC research creates a demand for embryonic stem cells

When discussing the use–derivation distinction, I argued that using embryonic stem cells is likely to encourage embryo destruction in several ways. One is by creating a demand for embryonic stem cells, thereby expectably increasing the supply of embryonic stem cell lines, and thus the number of embryos destroyed. Even if the additional demand created by an individual researcher will not in fact take the level of demand across the threshold necessary to have an effect on the supply, it cannot be ascertained in advance whether this is so, so it should be expected that the use of embryonic stem cells will expectably increase the number of embryos destroyed, and this is presumptively wrong (if embryo destruction is wrong).

There is, however, reason to believe that iPSC research, as it is currently done, also encourages embryo destruction through the creation of a demand, though perhaps in a more indirect way. Although the iPSC technique is very promising, it needs to be further developed. As mentioned earlier, this requires constant comparisons with embryonic stem cell research, which is still considered to be the gold standard.

However, it is not only the case that researchers should compare iPSCs with *existing* findings on embryonic stem cells; to make useful comparisons it is also important that embryonic stem cell research *continues*. For example, to investigate whether iPSCs are molecularly and functionally equivalent to embryonic stem cells, the latter need to be understood in much greater detail.[62]

Yamanaka, pioneer of iPSC research (and winner of the Nobel Prize in Physiology or Medicine 2012), writes:

ES cells are at least a few years more advanced than iPS cells in terms of safety. Therefore, preclinical and clinical trials using ES cells should be continued. A few years means a lot for patients who are urgently waiting for new treatments. I would expect that iPS cells will eventually replace ES cells in most, if not all, applications in the future. Even thereafter, however, ES cells are still expected to have an important role as a control in both experiments and trials.

---

[62] Daley et al., 'Broader Implications of Defining Standards for the Pluripotency of iPSCs'. Belmonte et al., 'Induced Pluripotent Stem Cells and Reprogramming'. Baker, 'iPS Cells: Potent Stuff'.

If the further development of the iPSC technique requires comparisons with ongoing embryonic stem cell research, it seems that iPSC researchers create a demand for such research and thereby encourage it.

There is another way in which iPSC research could create a demand for embryonic stem cell research, and thus for embryonic stem cells. Different methods of obtaining pluripotent stem cells may prove more useful for particular purposes. For example, suppose iPSC research is unable to solve a particular problem but shows that embryonic stem cell research likely would be able to solve it. Imagine a scenario where iPSCs are used in important biomedical research that may benefit patients with heart disease. However, it turns out that the final (but essential) step in the research process cannot be done using iPSCs. There are, however, good scientific reasons to think that embryonic stem cells are more promising candidates for doing the last step. This would create a strong incentive to do the relevant embryonic stem cell research: an incentive that would not have existed had the iPSC research not been done. This may also apply to therapeutic uses of iPSCs and embryonic stem cells. Doubts have been raised about the usefulness of iPSCs for therapy. But if iPSC research highlights that embryonic stem cells are likely to be promising for certain therapeutic uses, there will be a strong temptation to further pursue embryonic stem cell research.

It seems thus that iPSC research encourages embryonic stem cells research. If it does, then it also indirectly encourages embryo destruction. Thus, just like the use of embryonic stem cells in research, iPSC research raises thorny issues regarding indirect encouragement of embryo destruction. This is the second reason why iPSC research does not avoid the ethical problem of embryo destruction.[63]

Of course, one might object that these arguments could apply to adult stem cell research as well, and even to any other scientific research that indirectly encourages embryonic stem cell research in this way. But there is a difference. Unlike adult stem cells, iPSCs and embryonic stem cells are both pluripotent cells and, in the case of embryonic stem cells produced through SCNT, potentially patient-matched pluripotent stem cells. They are, therefore, regarded as much more complementary.[64] This

---

[63] Mark T. Brown, 'Moral Complicity in Induced Pluripotent Stem Cell Research', *Kennedy Institute of Ethics Journal*, 19 (2009), 1–22.

[64] Robinton and Daley, 'Promise of Induced Pluripotent Stem Cells'.

has resulted in much closer collaboration between researchers from both fields (embryonic stem cells research and iPSC research) than between researchers working with embryonic stem cells and adult stem cells. Indeed, often the same researchers conduct both iPSC and embryonic stem cell research.[65]

Thus, it is fair to say that embryonic stem cell and iPSC research progress in parallel and mutually support one another. Just like the use of already existing embryonic stem cells is likely to inspire and stimulate embryonic stem cell research in less restrictive countries where embryonic stem cell derivation is allowed, iPSC research is likely to inspire and stimulate embryonic stem cell research in countries where this research is allowed and supported.

iPSC research expresses support for embryonic stem cell research

We also saw in section 3.3 that using embryonic stem cells might reasonably be regarded as expressing support for embryo destruction, and this may also indirectly encourage embryo destruction. Researchers conducting research on embryonic stem cells are not only knowingly encouraging the production of embryonic stem cell lines, they are also closely cooperating with and sharing the aims of those deriving and supplying embryonic stem cells. Since they do not distance themselves from embryo destruction in any plausible way it is reasonable to assume they are, in fact, supporting, and thereby indirectly encouraging it. (Recall that we contrasted this with the Murder Victim case in which there was no reason to assume that the surgeon, or the patient, by benefiting from murder, encourages murder.)

However, can research with iPSCs reasonably be interpreted as expressing support for embryonic stem cell research? Surely iPSC researchers knowingly encourage embryonic stem cell research, but perhaps they can do this without expressing support for it? They might, for example, regret that their research encourages embryonic stem cell research, and justify this effect by the major benefits of iPSC research, one of which is that at some point in the future it may make embryonic stem cell research redundant.

---

[65] Scott et al., 'Democracy Derived?'.

Do researchers conducting iPSC research cooperate and share intentions with embryonic stem cell researchers? They currently rely heavily on knowledge gained in embryonic stem cell research, but that in itself is not sufficient for expressing support for embryonic stem cell research. If we use 'medical' data obtained by Nazis for important biomedical research we do not necessarily express support for the Nazi atrocities. We can avoid expressing support for these atrocities by clearly distancing ourselves from them, for example, by explicitly disapproving of these atrocities and by subjecting the use of data resulting from these atrocities to debate. It seems to me, however, that it is only possible to distance ourselves from the Nazi atrocities because they lie in the past. It would be an entirely different matter if the Nazis were still conducting their experiments.

Can researchers conducting iPSC research distance themselves from embryonic stem cell research? Since iPSC research relies so heavily on embryonic stem cells research, researchers working with iPSCs regularly cite embryonic stem cell research in their papers, without openly disapproving of such research. When researchers knowingly benefit from atrocious Nazi experiments, and cite these experiments, we generally expect them to explicitly state that they disapprove of the experiments. As mentioned earlier, researchers working with iPSCs also often closely collaborate with embryonic stem cell researchers; indeed, it is often the case that researchers interested in iPSC research also conduct or have conducted embryonic stem cell research themselves. Moreover, as Yamanaka's quotation illustrates, even the pioneers of iPSC research, who believe that iPSC research will one day replace embryonic stem cell research, stress that embryonic stem cell research should nevertheless continue for comparative research.

This suggests that for many scientists, the main motivation behind conducting iPSC research is that it is scientifically more promising, or that it is more efficient, easier, and cheaper than embryonic stem cell research, and that it avoids many of its administrative complexities. If iPSC researchers were motivated by a concern for embryos, laboratories working on iPSC research would, or at least should, avoid as much as possible any association with embryonic stem cell research. If iPSC scientists do not distance themselves from embryonic stem cell research, it seems plausible to assume they are in fact condoning such research.

For those who find embryonic stem cell research acceptable, the concerns about encouraging embryo destruction by conducting iPSC

research may be difficult to comprehend. But they could have great force
for those who are strongly opposed to embryonic stem cell research. This
can be brought out with the following hypothetical case.

> *Evil Operations.* Surgeons worldwide are working on a new surgical
> technique (NT) that could save many lives and reduce morbidity
> considerably. However, the most promising way to develop NT is
> through research on organs obtained through painful and fatal oper-
> ations on randomly chosen innocent people; the physiological effects
> of the torture on the organs provide crucial information for the
> research. Many people have lost their partners, friends, and family
> members this way and everyone is constantly worried about who will be
> selected next. Some think the benefits outweigh the harms, but many
> think that the operations are evil, and that those using the organs to test
> NT act wrongly because they encourage this evil. Fortunately, a group of
> surgeons has developed a new method for testing NT that does not
> require the horrific operations; instead, computer simulations are used.
> Surgeons using the computer simulations closely collaborate with sur-
> geons removing and using the organs, as this method is still considered
> the most efficient method to further develop NT. Moreover, there is
> growing consensus that the organ and computer simulation methods
> are complementary, which gives surgeons even more reason to collab-
> orate and promote one another's work. Both methods mutually support
> each other. The government and people who think the operations are a
> great evil are happy with the development of the computer-simulated
> technique for perfecting NT. So happy that they ignore or remain silent
> on its close association with the ongoing evil operations.

Regarding this case, we would be inclined to say that those working on
the computer-simulated technique act wrongly because they encourage
the organ research, and that those doing research on the organs encourage the evil operations via which they are obtained. But for those who
think destroying embryos is as wicked as the operations, embryonic stem
cell research is analogous to the organ research in this case, while iPSC
research is analogous to the computer-simulation research.[66]

---

[66] There is, of course, one disanalogy between the iPSC case and Evil Operations. In the
latter, people are constantly worried about who will be selected next, whereas something
similar would not be the case for embryo destruction. However, with Evil Operations,

The interconnectedness of iPSC and embryonic stem cell research

The connections between iPSC and embryonic stem cell research are similar to the connections between embryonic stem cell research and embryo destruction. Research on embryonic stem cells arguably encourages embryo destruction through increasing the demand for embryonic stem cell lines; similarly iPSC research arguably promotes embryonic stem cell research in the same way. Engaging in embryonic stem cell research arguably also implicitly condones embryo destruction, in part because it involves significant interaction with those who destroy embryos. Engaging in iPSC research also involves significant interaction with embryonic stem cell researchers—indeed often iPSC researchers conduct embryonic stem cell research themselves—and thus, plausibly, also implicitly condone embryonic stem cell research, thereby indirectly encouraging embryo destruction.

Given that the connections between research using embryonic stem cells and embryo destruction and iPSC research and embryo destruction are similar, it is difficult to see how those who oppose embryonic stem cell research on the grounds that it encourages wrongful embryo destruction can escape the conclusion that engaging in iPSC research is also wrong. Consistency requires that considerations regarding encouragement of embryo destruction are invoked in both cases. There seem, then, to be three options.

First, one could reject both embryonic stem cell research and iPSC research on the basis that both types of research encourage embryo destruction. This option is, however, unappealing given the immense promises of both types of research.

A second option would be to advocate a change in the ways iPSC research is done so that it would no longer encourage embryonic stem cell research. However, this option is equally unappealing. It would not only considerably slow down iPSC research. It would also make it much more unlikely that the goals of iPSC research will actually be achieved.

I merely mean to give an example of a practice that many would consider obviously wrong, so as to better understand how those believing an embryo is a person could evaluate the connection between iPSC research and embryonic stem cell research.

Third, one could seek some principled basis for thinking that encouraging embryo destruction by conducting embryonic stem cell research is significantly worse than encouraging embryo destruction by conducting iPSC research. For example, it could be argued that it is encouraging wrongdoing through softening our attitudes that is most important. This softening of attitudes seems to be a genuine possibility in the case of embryonic stem cell research, but may be less of a concern in the case of iPSC research.

Of course, there is another possibility for rejecting arguments referring to the encouragement of embryo destruction against both iPSC and embryonic stem cell research. One could deny that destroying early embryos for important scientific research is wrong. If destroying embryos for important scientific research is permissible, then there is nothing wrong with encouraging it. Both embryonic stem cell research and iPSC research would then be permissible.

In any case, that iPSC research indirectly encourages embryo destruction is the second reason why the embryonic stem cell debate is not over yet. I will now briefly discuss the third reason.

Are induced pluripotent stem cells potential babies?

In July 2009, two research groups independently reported the first successful generation of adult mice from iPSCs via tetraploid complementation.[67] These experiments are part of ongoing research into the differences and similarities between iPSCs and embryonic stem cells. If iPSCs are found to be similar to embryonic stem cells in terms of their ability to differentiate into any cell type, this will more likely make the use of the latter in research redundant in the long term. Thus, the tetraploid complementation experiments raise the hopes of those who oppose embryonic stem cell research and want to see it replaced by iPSC research. However, the very same research creates ethical challenges for them. Similarities between iPSCs and embryonic stem cells cast doubt on one of the main arguments against embryonic stem cell research: that it is wrong to destroy an embryo because it has the potential to become a person.

---

[67] Lan Kang et al., 'iPS Cells Can Support Full-Term Development of Tetraploid Blastocyst-Complemented Embryos', *Cell Stem Cell,* 5 (2009), 135–8. Xiao-yang Zhao et al., 'iPS Cells Produce Viable Mice through Tetraploid Complementation', *Nature,* 461 (2009), 86–90.

In section 3.2, I argued that tetraploid complementation experiments in the mouse suggest that embryonic stem cells have very similar potential to that of embryos. For those who accord a significant moral status to the early embryo in virtue of its potential to become a person, this raises an interesting dilemma: they must either treat embryonic stem cells as morally significant entities worthy of protection and thus oppose the use of embryonic stem cells, or admit that early embryos do not derive their significant moral status from the potential they possess, and thus reject the potentiality argument.

Since 2009, we know that iPSCs can also give rise to a full-grown organism when complemented with a surrogate trophoblast. This suggests that iPSCs too may have the potential to become a person when placed in an appropriate environment.[68] The dilemma opponents of embryo research who accept the potentiality argument are confronted with thus extends to iPSC research: if they continue to appeal to the potentiality argument, they also risk undermining the use of iPSCs for research. Alternatively, if they reject the potentiality argument, they must eschew restrictions on embryo research or seek some other basis for them.

4.5. Conclusion

Some have suggested that if embryonic stem cells, or their functional equivalents, could be created without destroying embryos, a good deal of the ethical controversy surrounding embryonic stem cell research would subside and the Problem would dissolve. This resulted in a growing trend to seek technical solutions to the problem of destroying embryos to obtain stem cells. I have tried to show that the proposed solutions not only face serious scientific and technical challenges, suggesting that if used as the sole source of pluripotent stem cells, the rate of progress in stem cell research would be dramatically retarded, they also fail to avoid the problem of embryo destruction. The proposal to use organismically dead embryos as a source of stem cells raises concerns about the concept 'organismic death'. Organismically dead embryos might be more akin to severely disabled people than to brain-dead people, making it

---

[68]   Denker, 'Induced Pluripotent Stem Cells'.

problematic to destroy them for research. The use of organismically dead embryos also involves benefiting from, and thus encouraging, woman-friendly IVF. Blastomere biopsy is mainly problematic because the biopsied blastomere could be totipotent, and thus in fact an embryo. The blastocyst transfer method avoids this problem but faces other challenges because both its development and its application expose the embryo to significant harm, and it is not clear how this harm can be outweighed by any benefits for the embryo. The creation of biological artefacts through altered nuclear transfer, whether by altering Cdx2 or Nanog, is problematic because it is plausible to regard ANTities as normal embryos programmed for an early death, or as disabled embryos. Parthenogenesis raises similar questions about the moral status of parthenotes. Many believe that parthenotes are embryos as they can develop normally up to the blastocyst stage. Thus, the proposed alternatives for obtaining pluripotent stem cells without harming embryos do not offer a satisfactory solution to the Problem.

The iPSC technique has raised the highest hopes for putting an end to the embryonic stem cell debate. I have, however, argued that iPSC research does not provide a solution to the Problem, at least not at this point in time. First, scientific research suggests that iPSC research cannot replace embryonic stem cell research in the near or mid-term future. Second, iPSC research is extremely closely intertwined with embryonic stem cell research. The further development of iPSC research requires constant comparisons with past, current, and future embryonic stem cell research, thereby creating a demand for such research. Researchers conducting iPSC research may also indirectly encourage embryonic stem cell research by expressing support for it. Thus, iPSC cell research encourages embryonic stem cell research, and thus, indirectly, embryo destruction and this is presumptively wrong if the embryo has a significant moral status. A third reason why iPSC research may not mark the end of the embryonic stem cell debate is that iPSCs, just like embryonic stem cells, seem to have the potential to become a person. This challenges the view that it is wrong to destroy embryos because they are potential persons.

5
Compromise and Consistency

5.1. Consistency

Before I outline some implications and draw a few conclusions, let me first briefly summarize what I have tried to show in this book.

Summary

The focus of the book has been on the two main types of response to the Problem, which I outlined in Chapter 1. The Problem is that either one supports embryonic stem cell research and accepts resulting embryo destruction, or one opposes embryonic stem cell research and accepts that the potential benefits of this research will be foregone.

What is important is that those who accord a significant moral status to the embryo—either a full moral status or a high intermediate moral status—have tried to look for a solution to the Problem without having to modify their view on the embryo's moral status. The first type of response has been to develop a middle-ground position, a position intermediate between the dominant opposing views on the permissibility of embryonic stem cell research. In Chapter 2, I discussed one such position, the discarded–created distinction, which holds that using and deriving stem cells from discarded embryos is presumptively permissible, but using and deriving stem cells from research embryos is not. I argued that none of the arguments adduced in support of the discarded–created distinction could justify the view that it is significantly worse to use and derive stem cells from research embryos than to use and derive stem cells from discarded embryos. The expected benefits of the two different kinds of research are both very large, and there does not seem to be a significant difference in the moral costs. Thus, if one accepts the derivation of stem cells from discarded embryos, consistency requires that one also accept the derivation of stem cells from research embryos. In Chapter 3,

I investigated a second middle-ground position: the use–derivation distinction. This position holds that it may be permissible to use embryonic stem cells but it is never permissible to derive them, since this involves embryo destruction. An assumption underlying this position is that embryonic stem cells are neither embryos nor their moral equivalents. I argued that tetraploid complementation experiments cast doubt on this assumption, at least if one accords a moral status to the embryo in virtue of its potential to develop into a person. I then considered the main defence of the use–derivation distinction. This appeals to the view that using embryonic stem cells does not encourage embryo destruction. I argued that, by using embryonic stem cells, a researcher always directly or indirectly encourages embryo destruction in a way that makes it presumptively wrong. She does so either by (expectably) pushing the demand over or closer to the threshold required to increase the supply of embryonic stem cell lines, or by being part of a group that does so. I concluded that, as long as no stronger arguments are presented in support of the use–derivation distinction, we should reject it. Either one should accept both the use and derivation of embryonic stem cells, or neither.

In Chapter 4, I discussed the second type of response to the Problem: the development of technical solutions that allow scientists to obtain embryonic stem cells, or their functional equivalents, but without harming embryos. I first evaluated the use of organismically dead embryos, blastomere biopsy, the blastocyst transfer method, altered nuclear transfer (ANT), and parthenogenesis. All of these proposed solutions face serious scientific and technical challenges so that using them as the sole source of embryos would severely restrict scientific and medical progress. More importantly, however, they fail to avoid the problem of embryo destruction. Each proposed technique results in harm to or destruction of embryos, or would rely on other research that does so.

The induced pluripotent stem cell technique has raised the highest hopes for ending the embryonic stem cell debate, but it too fails to offer a complete solution to the Problem. First, iPSC research is unlikely to replace embryonic stem cell research in the near or mid-term future. Second, iPSC research is so dependent on (the continuation of) embryonic stem cell research that it in fact encourages such research, and thus embryo destruction. The position holding that it is permissible to conduct iPSC research but impermissible to conduct embryonic stem cell research is, like the discarded–created and the use–derivation distinctions, inconsistent. (Note that if one accepts iPSC research one implicitly endorses embryonic stem cell research, and thus one implicitly adopts a kind of middle-ground position, even if one explicitly maintains that embryonic stem cell research is impermissible.)

All of the positions that I have been arguing against fail for similar reasons: they depend on inconsistent argumentation. In each case, either (i) the argument that the supposedly permissible kind of research is permissible also shows that the supposedly impermissible kind of research is permissible, or (ii) the argument that the supposedly impermissible kind of research is impermissible also shows that the supposedly permissible kind of research is impermissible. The arguments for these positions only appear to succeed if we apply those arguments selectively to certain types of pluripotent stem cell research, without drawing out their implications for others.

The slide to the ultimate wrongdoing

My arguments seem to have a shocking implication. What I have tried to show is that iPSC research, as it is currently done, encourages embryonic stem cell research. Furthermore, embryonic stem cell research encourages the generation of embryonic stem cells, and thus the destruction of discarded embryos. Moreover, the destruction of discarded embryos is not significantly morally different from the destruction of research embryos. Both directly or indirectly encourage the creation of embryos that are (likely to be) destined to be destroyed for beneficial purposes. Though a researcher who engages in iPSC cell research is rather removed from the actual creation and destruction of embryos, I have argued that none of the commonly suggested points on the spectrum between performing iPSC research and creating or destroying research embryos marks a morally significant difference such that it can be argued that research on one side of the cut-off point is permissible, and research on the other is not. Do we have to conclude, then, that if one believes that iPSC research is presumptively permissible one is committed to finding the creation and destruction of research embryos also presumptively permissible?

That seems implausible. However, if my arguments have been sound, it is now up to the defenders of the middle-ground positions to come up with convincing arguments to show why the slide from accepting iPSC research to accepting the creation and destruction of research embryos does not occur.

Perhaps the most plausible approach would be to construct an argument that appeals to the moral relevance of the researcher's causal proximity to the wrongdoing. It could perhaps be argued that each action on the chain from embryo creation and destruction to the carrying out of iPSC research is somewhat more removed, causally, from what those who accord a significant moral status to the embryo consider to be the ultimate wrongdoing. The idea would then be that the more removed from the ultimate wrongdoing, the less morally problematic one's action is.

Thus, one could maintain that using iPSCs is somewhat less problematic than using embryonic stem cells because, even though it encourages embryo destruction, it is less causally proximate to that destruction than is using embryonic stem cells. Likewise one could hold that, even though using embryonic stem cells encourages embryo destruction, this is less problematic than destroying the embryos oneself. The causal path to the wrongdoing is longer. Finally, one could argue that destroying discarded embryos is less problematic than destroying research embryos because the encouragement of the wrongdoing—the creation of embryos destined to die for beneficial purposes—is causally more remote. We could call this the 'causal distance' argument.[1]

Which of the moral lines drawn by the various middle-ground positions one chooses will then partly depend on how much one thinks causal distance attenuates one's reasons to abstain from research, as well as on exactly what moral status one accords to the embryo. Those who accord a very high intermediate moral status to the embryo are more likely to support the moral distinction between iPSC and embryonic stem cell research, those who accord a somewhat lower moral status may rather choose the use–derivation distinction, and those who accord a low intermediate moral status to the embryo might opt for the discarded–created distinction.

---

[1] An alternative argument could refer to the indirectness of the wrongdoing. It could be argued that the more indirect one's connection is to the ultimate wrongdoing (i.e. the more other agents are involved as intermediaries), the less problematic one's action is. If one thinks indirectness and not causal distance is what matters, then one could read 'causal distance' as referring to 'indirectness' in this section.

However, to make the causal distance argument work, the defenders of the middle-ground positions would have to overcome another challenge. According to the causal distance argument, each time we add a more controversial aspect or type of stem cell research to what is already considered permissible by the middle-ground position in question (for example, we add research on already existing embryonic stem cells to iPSC research, or stem cell derivation from discarded embryos to research on already existing embryonic stem cells) there is an extra moral cost. This is because there has been a qualitative change in the research; it has moved closer, in causal terms, to the creation and destruction of embryos for the purpose of research. However, each time we add a more controversial aspect or type of research, we also gain a significant benefit. This is because the expected benefits of, for example, conducting iPSC research *and* embryonic stem cell research are *significantly* greater than the benefits of conducting iPSC research alone. Adding this more controversial type of research to iPSC research not only allows new applications that require embryonic stem cells, but also significantly contributes to iPSC research. Likewise, the benefits of research on iPSCs and embryonic stem cells *and* of deriving embryonic stem cells are *significantly* greater than the benefits of merely conducting research on embryonic stem cells and iPSCs, and so forth. What defenders of the middle-ground positions need to show then is that, for at least one more controversial aspect or type of stem cell research, the increase in moral cost associated with adding that aspect or type of research is greater than the increase in benefits, so that, overall, adding it is a morally bad thing to do. They must show that the fact the researcher's action moves somewhat closer, in a causal terms, to the ultimate wrongdoing increases the moral cost to such an extent that it can no longer be outweighed by the significant increase in benefits that will occur by adding that controversial aspect or type of research. It is not clear whether such an argument will be convincing. Thus, in the absence of a further argument, these positions remain plagued by inconsistency in the sense I described. This might seem to be a fatal problem: surely we should never defend inconsistent ethical positions. Or should we?

5.2. Compromise

My focus up until now has been on the quality of the main arguments adduced in support of the ethical positions that try to offer a solution to the Problem. The arguments I have been criticizing were intended to show that these positions are the correct ethical positions—that they correctly described the permissibility and impermissibility of different types or aspects of stem cell research. I have tried to show that these arguments are unconvincing, for example, because they are inherently inconsistent or have been inconsistently applied, and that, as a result, the ethical positions they are meant to support are not correct—they are not true or epistemically justified. But I have been silent on the argument that, even if these positions are not the correct ethical positions, we might still have strong reasons to publicly defend or accept them, for example, because this will have the best consequences, or because this expresses respect for a variety of reasonable views in a democratic society.

Thus, perhaps one could agree that the middle-ground positions or the scientific solutions are inconsistent, and thus presumably incorrect, but argue that we should treat them as correct for the purposes of making policy, or perhaps even for the purposes of engaging in public debate about stem cell research. One may argue that the fact that these positions are inconsistent does not provide an all-things-considered reason not to defend them or build stem cell policy around them. The idea is that the inconsistency of the arguments underlying these positions only provides *one* reason not to defend them as an ethical basis for stem cell policy. There could be stronger countervailing reasons in favour of defending them.

Heidi Mertes and Guido Pennings, for example, have argued that it is not only permissible, but sometimes even morally obligatory, for countries to base their stem cell policy on a middle-ground position, even 'if it does not represent a solid moral conviction'.[2] They acknowledge, for example, that the use–derivation distinction is an inconsistent ethical position but they believe that countries should nevertheless defend it as a compromise.

This raises an important question that I have ignored so far. Should one defend any of the middle-ground positions or technical solutions in the embryonic stem cell debate as a compromise position? I do not intend to give a conclusive answer to this question here. However, I would like to draw out some reasons for and against doing so.[3]

---

[2] Heidi Mertes and Guido Pennings, 'Stem Cell Research Policies: Who's Afraid of Complicity?', *Reproductive BioMedicine Online*, 19 (2009), 38–42.

[3] The analysis of reasons for and against compromise in this chapter are based on a manuscript that Thomas Douglas and I wrote together entitled 'The Epistemic Costs of Compromise in Ethical Debate'.

When is a middle-ground position a compromise?

One can defend a middle-ground position in the embryonic stem cell debate because one thinks it is the true or epistemically justified (henceforth collectively 'correct') ethical position, regardless of whether it is intermediate between the position that all and no embryonic stem cell research is permissible. It might then just be a coincidence that the position one defends is a position between more obvious or dominant opposing views. So far, I have been dealing with the middle-ground positions and technical solutions as positions that have been defended simply because they are believed to be correct.

However, sometimes when one defends a middle-ground position one defends that position in part *because* it is intermediate between opposing views. Indeed, the use–derivation and discarded–created distinctions are sometimes in part defended *because* they are positions intermediate between the views that all and no embryonic stem cell research is permissible. The same is true for the technical solutions—they have also sometimes been defended, not because they are believed to be the correct positions, but because they are intermediate between opposing views on the ethics of embryonic stem cell research. One could say then that in such cases the technical solutions are defended as middle-ground positions.

Why would one defend a position *because* it is a position between more obvious or dominant opposing views? One could have epistemic or practical reasons to do so.

One would have epistemic reasons to do so when the fact that the position lies in between more obvious or dominant positions gives one *evidence* for the position. For example, one may believe that it may make the position more likely to be correct. Indeed, the presence of contrasting dominant views may count as evidence for the fact that the correct position lies somewhere in between. For example, it seems plausible that, for many who adopt the intermediate moral status view on the embryo, at least part of the motivation for adopting this view is the thought that, when a significant number of people have strong, and strongly opposing views on this matter (the embryo has no or a full moral status), the truth must lie somewhere in between. Perhaps some have adopted the use–derivation or the discarded–created distinction for the same reason. However, if one acknowledges that the middle-ground position one defends is inconsistent (as Mertes and Pennings do) then one's reasons for adopting it are unlikely to be epistemic reasons, for it is normally thought that, where, following careful reflection, one can argue for a position only by applying arguments inconsistently, we have strong evidence against the correctness of the position.

In that case one may take the middle ground for *practical* reasons. These can be moral or prudential. One can take the middle ground because this will have good consequences for oneself. For example, one can take the middle ground in order to acquire more political influence and thus advance one's career, in order to appear reasonable and thus garner the admiration of others, or in order to avoid the discomfort of facing strong disagreement from others. In such cases, one takes the middle ground for prudential reasons.

Moral reasons for taking the middle ground would include a concern to advance the public good. It has been argued that when ethicists take part in the policy-making process, for example, by serving on an ethics committee, they should act with the public good in mind.[4] Suppose an ethicist is asked to advise on organ transplantation policy. The ethicist believes that organ conscription from deceased individuals is permissible—she believes it is morally permissible to transplant organs from deceased persons regardless of their wishes or decisions when living. But suppose that the current policy permits organs to be transplanted only when the deceased individual previously actively consented to this. The ethicist might then defend a weaker view than her own, such as that it is morally permissible to transplant organs when consent can reasonably be presumed, but not otherwise. She might defend this weaker view on the grounds that it is much more likely to be accepted and enacted in policy, and that the number of organ transplants thereby foregone, compared to enacting a policy of organ conscription, would be small. If she defended her true, more extreme view, she might lose credibility, and this might reduce the chance of any deviation from the status quo being accepted, resulting in worse consequences for society (in this case, fewer organ transplants). The ethicist defends the middle ground *not* because it is likely to be correct, nor for prudential reasons,

---

[4] Dan W. Brock, 'Truth or Consequences: The Role of Philosophers in Policy-Making', *Ethics*, 97 (1987), 787.

but for moral reasons, in this case, instrumental moral reasons: she defends it in order to promote the public good.

In the stem cell debate too, ethicists serving on an ethics committee may defend a middle-ground position. They might, for example, defend the discarded–created distinction because if they defended the position they really believe to be true (for example, that there is no reason to consider destroying research embryos as morally worse than destroying discarded embryos) they might lose their credibility, and this may result in a more restrictive position than the discarded–created distinction being adopted, which, arguably, would be detrimental to the public good.

One might have various other instrumental moral reasons to take the middle ground. For example, one may believe it to be the best available option to increase social solidarity, prevent paralytic disagreement, lead to the selection of the best feasible policy alternative (the policy that enacts the correct ethical position may be infeasible), or trigger a stepwise progression such that protagonists to the debate will arrive at the correct position in the long run. In all these cases, taking the middle ground is a means to the end of advancing the public good or some impersonal good—perhaps fairness, virtue, achievement, and knowledge.

Alternatively, one could have non-instrumental moral reasons to take the middle ground. For example, one may take the middle ground as doing so might appropriately respect the reasonable views taken by others. One may believe that adherents of the full and no moral status views have sincerely adopted reasonable moral positions on the permissibility of embryonic stem cell research, and that their views ought to be respected. One may believe that adopting a middle-ground position on the morality of embryonic stem cell research maximally respects those views. Taking the middle ground is not done for instrumental reasons in this case. It is not that taking the middle ground causes some further goal to be realized. Rather, taking the middle ground is constitutive of respecting the views of others, which is taken to be valuable, or morally required, in itself.

Mertes and Pennings, for example, have argued that it is perfectly acceptable to defend the use–derivation distinction on the ground that it maximally respects the conflicting moral values within a morally divided society. According to Mertes and Pennings one has a moral obligation to defend what they refer to as a 'principled compromise':

[T]here is no reason why a country should only strive for 'maximal innocence' with regard to embryo destruction. On the contrary, there is a moral obligation to search for a position that maximally respects the conflicting moral values: in this case, respect for the embryos and the development of cures for debilitating diseases. A compromise position that allows certain aspects of human ESC research while avoiding the core characteristics of moral complicity to embryo destruction (by not intentionally causing it) is therefore an acceptable position.[5]

Finally, one could have character-based moral reasons for taking the middle ground. Refusing to shift one's view in the face of disagreement closer to that of others may express aggressiveness or dogmatism, whereas accommodating one's views to those of others may express tolerance, humility, and modesty. Arthur Kuflik, for example, has argued that compromise often manifests 'a love for peace and a distaste for fanaticism'.[6] On some views, the fact that defending a middle-ground position would manifest or express admirable character traits could give one a moral reason to do it.

I reserve the term 'compromise position' for a middle-ground position that one defends for practical reasons even though one believes that epistemic reasons militate against doing so. On this way of thinking, one can acknowledge that the use–derivation or discarded–created distinctions or the technical solutions are inconsistent, but nevertheless defend them for practical reasons, that is, as compromises.

Perhaps there are moral reasons to defend the middle-ground positions in the stem cell debate as compromises. However, what has typically been ignored in that debate is that even if this is so, there is also almost always a cost attached to defending a compromise. This makes compromises almost always problematic to some degree. Even though this does not mean that compromise is always wrong, it *does* provide a reason against compromising that should be taken into account when one deliberates about whether or not to defend a compromise. Moreover, even when, in the end, one decides to defend a compromise (because the reasons for outweigh the reasons against doing so), one may still be able to reduce the cost attached to it.

But what is this cost I have in mind? Why is compromise almost always problematic?

---

[5] Mertes and Pennings, 'Stem Cell Research Policies', 42.

[6] In David Braybrooke, 'The Possibilities of Compromise', *Ethics*, 93 (1982), 142.

The cost of compromises

The view that there is almost always something problematic about a compromise is in fact a widespread one. Several reasons are commonly cited for why this is so. I just mention the most common ones.

COWARDICE, HYPOCRISY, OR A LACK OF INTEGRITY

One explanation for why compromise is almost always problematic holds that it involves or expresses cowardice, hypocrisy, or a lack of integrity. These concepts are not easily definable, but usually the basic thought is that when one compromises one fails to stand up for one's core or authentic values.

Some compromises may indeed be problematic for this reason. For example, suppose someone committed to defending the truth without exception defends a view which he knows to be false. Or suppose someone committed to the moral equality of all persons compromises with someone who believes women are morally inferior. In these cases, the person may give up on one of her core commitments, and may thus act hypocritically or lose her integrity. However, in many cases, those who compromise do not give up on any core value. They may have no core commitment to defending the truth, or maintaining opposition to whomever they are arguing against. Moreover, if the value served by the compromise (for example, a commitment to seeking public agreement, or to advancing the public good) is itself a core value, it is not clear why sacrificing some other core value should involve a loss of integrity, hypocrisy, or cowardice. Indeed, sometimes defending a compromise may be necessary to preserve integrity, or to avoid hypocrisy or coward- ice. According to Mertes and Pennings, for example, countries that need to decide about what embryonic stem cell policy to implement must sometimes compromise in order to *avoid* being hypocritical.[7] Suppose that a country defends the view that an embryo has full moral status and should never be destroyed for research, but is also strongly committed to promoting medical research that could save and improve many lives. One could say that the country has two conflicting core commitments. Mertes and Pennings argue that the country should not go 'through extremes' to follow through on just one of these commitments at the cost

---

[7] Mertes and Pennings, 'Stem Cell Research Policies'.

of the other, since that would be hypocritical—it would imply that one gives up on a core commitment. The country should instead find a middle ground between fulfilling both commitments, for example, by allowing limited embryonic stem cell research.

Thus, there are cases where compromising does not involve a loss of integrity, hypocrisy, or cowardice. This suggests that compromise is not always problematic for this reason.

DECEPTION OR BAD FAITH

Another reason why compromise may be problematic is because it involves deception or bad faith. In some cases, a compromise will only serve its purpose when the resulting position is falsely presented as a position adopted for epistemic reasons, or at least where the practical reasons for defending the position are not expressed.

Dan Brock has described an instance of this problem, which he faced as a member of the professional staff of the President's Commission for the Study of Ethical Problems in Medicine.[8] When assigned to write a report representing the Commission's position on decisions about life-sustaining treatment, Brock had to decide about whether to press his own view on the killing/letting die distinction, which was that the distinction is not morally relevant. Many commissioners believed that killing was much more wrong than allowing to die and that stopping life support was a case of allowing to die, and thus permissible. Both Brock and the commissioners thought that it was permissible to stop life support upon the patient's request but the reasons they gave were different. If Brock tried to convince them of what he thought to be the right reasons then there was a risk that the commissioners would no longer support stopping life support on the patient's request, since they would realize this is morally equivalent to killing. To maximize the chance that withdrawal of life support would be tolerated, Brock chose to present his expressed view—that this was permissible because it was a case of allowing to die—as being defended for purely epistemic reasons. He had to conceal the fact that he thought the real reason for allowing it was that it might be permissible to kill a person, since revealing this

---

[8] Brock, 'Truth or Consequences'.

might have led the commissioners to change their position to a more prohibitive one.

There are some cases in which compromise positions will only achieve their intended purpose if there is an element of deception involved. However, compromise *need* not involve deception, and in some cases can achieve its goals even if explicitly presented for what it is. In those cases, one can compromise and be fully transparent about one's reasons for adopting the compromise position while still achieving one's practical goal.

Thus, appealing to deception alone cannot justify the view that there is almost always something problematic with compromise, since again compromise need not, and often does not, involve deception.

COMPLICITY

A third possible explanation for the problematic nature of compromise holds that it makes the compromiser complicit in maintaining one of the positions which the compromise seeks to accommodate—that is, one of the positions between which one seeks a middle ground. So, for example, if one is a liberal egalitarian and defends a compromise between the views of a liberal egalitarianism and anti-Semitism, one may become complicit in anti-Semitism, either in the sense that one causally contributes to its popularity, or in the sense that one implicitly condones it by treating it as a legitimate view.

Again, this explanation may show why some compromises are problematic, but many compromises remain untouched. Suppose one compromises with an anti-Semite precisely because one rightly believes that doing so is what will, in the long run, best undermine anti-Semitism. In this case, one is not complicit in anti-Semitism in the sense that one is causally contributing to it, and it is hard to see how one is complicit in the sense that one is treating it as a legitimate view. Many actual compromises in bioethics in fact seem to have precisely this form. For example, someone committed to both treatment withdrawal and active euthanasia for patients in a persistent vegetative state (PVS) may compromise with someone who believes patients in PVS should be kept alive, by holding that treatment withdrawal is permissible, but active euthanasia is not. He may do so precisely because he thinks that this is what will, in the end, best foster support for active euthanasia. He may reason that, if his opponents accept the compromise, this will make it more likely that they will, at some point in the future, be more willing to accept active euthanasia.

In sum, although defending a compromise may be problematic if it involves cowardice, lack of integrity, hypocrisy, deception, or complicity, in many cases defending a compromise is not problematic for any of these reasons. These explanations thus leave us a long way short of justifying the view according to which defending a compromise is almost always problematic. Why is it then that compromise is almost always problematic?

The epistemic cost of compromises

I believe that a better explanation for why compromising in ethics is almost always problematic appeals to the indirect epistemic costs of compromise. It seems that defending a compromise will typically make it more difficult to form correct—that is, true or epistemically justified—ethical beliefs in the future. There are at least two different ways in which compromise may do this. First, it may hamper the formation of correct beliefs by interfering with attempts to use the ethical beliefs of others as evidence. Let us call this the Problem of False Testimony. Second, it may weaken commitments important for epistemic progress. Let us call this the Problem of the Erosion of Epistemic Standards.

THE PROBLEM OF FALSE TESTIMONY

We often take the ethical claims of others as evidence for the correctness of these claims, much as we take the predictions of well-trained meteor-ologists as evidence for what the weather will be. For example, arguments in ethics often start from premises that are simply assumed to be correct because they are widely held, or (widely) held by serious ethicists. Similarly, policy-makers and practitioners who do not have the time to engage in ethical argument themselves may simply take a position to be correct or likely to be correct merely because it is a popular view, or a popular view among individuals deemed to be experts on the matter in question.

In many cases, this may be a rational thing to do, but in other cases it may not be. It would seem inappropriate when the popular position in question is a compromise position. These middle-ground positions are defended for practical reasons, which are not directly relevant to their correctness. Surely we would not take the predictions of rain made by meteorologists to have evidential value if we knew they only made the predictions to keep farmers happy, not on the basis of the meteorological evidence.

One problem with compromise positions in ethical debate, then, is that they are liable to be mistaken as having evidential value they in fact lack. This is especially the case when compromise positions are 'disguised', that is, when they are presented as middle-ground positions defended for epistemic reasons (as was the case in the anecdote discussed by Brock). But compromises can also be mistaken as having evidential value they in fact lack when they are *not* disguised. It may be that the practical reasons for defending a middle-ground position are initially disclosed, but, after a few iterations of discussion, are forgotten, for example, because the original reasons for defending the position are not always cited or correctly represented. Ethical positions often remain salient in ethical discussions long after the reasons for which they were defended are forgotten. If a compromise position is mistakenly taken to have evidential value it in fact lacks, this has an epistemically corrupting effect on the debate, and thus on regulations resulting from the debate.

The presence of compromises in the ethical literature, disguised or not, reduces the evidential value of that literature and hinders the formation of correct beliefs.

THE PROBLEM OF THE EROSION OF EPISTEMIC STANDARDS

A second way in which compromise may undermine the epistemic function of ethical debate is by weakening certain commitments that are important for epistemic progress in ethics.

How might compromising weaken these commitments? It is plausible to think that, in general, compromise positions will tend to lack certain virtues that positions defended because they are thought to be correct will possess: these virtues—epistemic virtues—may include simplicity and internal consistency, both features that are often thought to characterize correct moral positions. Since compromise positions are not defended because of their correctness, we might expect them to be, on average, more complex and less internally consistent than other positions defended in ethics. I have shown how this is the case with the middle-ground positions defended in the embryonic stem cell debate.

Taken on its own, the relative lack of epistemic virtue in compromise positions might be thought unproblematic: compromise positions are not defended because they are true or epistemically justified, so it is not clear why they need to possess features such as simplicity and internal consistency. The lack of epistemic virtues in compromise positions only becomes a problem because compromise positions are often mistakenly taken to be positions defended because of their (likely) correctness. As mentioned earlier, even when positions are explicitly presented as compromise positions by their proponents, their status as compromise positions is frequently forgotten after several iterations of debate. This can create a situation in which a debate or body of literature is populated by a number of positions, all of which are taken to be positions defended for their correctness, but only some of which were in fact defended for this reason. Those positions that were not defended for their correctness, but were rather defended as compromise positions, can be expected to lack epistemic virtues such as simplicity and internal consistency. Their presence in the literature will thus tend to drag down the average epistemic quality of the debate. To someone who enters the debate and is unaware of the fact that many of the positions defended therein were defended as compromises, it may simply appear as if the protagonists in the debate have been aiming to develop correct positions, but have not been very effective at doing so. Alternatively, it may appear that the protagonists in the debate are confused about what the epistemic standards are they should be applying. Either way, the result may be that the newcomer also adopts low epistemic standards, or forms no clear view on what epistemic standards she should be aiming for.

By analogy, consider a case in which a number of people are playing football in a park and a new potential player appears on the scene. Suppose that some of the players are playing to win, while others are playing in a non-competitive fashion, and are merely seeking to spend a relaxing afternoon in the park. These latter players are not, unsurprisingly, playing to a very high standard. If the newcomer thinks that all of the players are doing their best, she may simply come to the conclusion that the average standard of football being played is low, and this might lead her to set low standards for her own play as well.

Similar phenomena may occur in ethical debates: the failure to recognize compromise positions as such may lead either to a lowering of epistemic standards, or to general confusion about what the epistemic standards are.

I think, then, that compromise will typically have two epistemic costs. It will corrupt attempts to take the claims of ethicists as evidence for the correctness of those claims, and it will undermine standards that are important to making epistemic progress in ethics. Importantly, it does not follow from this that the epistemic cost always outweighs the moral benefits of defending compromise positions (for example, the fact that it would maximally respect the widely divergent views that people have on stem cell ethics), which can be significant. My argument only suggests that compromise is typically in one way problematic and that one therefore needs a good reason to accept or defend a compromise rather than accepting or defending what one believes to be the correct ethical position.

It seems that almost all compromises will have one or the other of these costs to at least some extent and that this explanation thus vindicates the view that compromise is almost always problematic. In particular, this explanation seems able to account for the problematic nature of compromises, even of transparent compromises, since even if one is open about one's practical reasons for taking the middle ground, there will typically still be a significant risk that, in subsequent debate, one's reasons for taking the middle ground will be forgotten. It is this subsequent failure on the part of others to recognize compromise positions for what they are that creates both the Problem of False Testimony and the Problem of Erosion of Epistemic Standards.

5.3. Compromise and Consistency in the Embryonic Stem Cell Debate

Since it was not the aim of this book to directly provide policy advice, it was an easy choice for me to write it in 'epistemic mode'. I have focused on the truth or coherence of the positions, and particularly on the consistency of arguments said to support them, rather than on the practical reasons for defending them. Had I instead been writing a report for the government, and thus in 'advisory mode', I may have reached different conclusions about the positions discussed. This would depend on the circumstances.

However, I do want to point out that what is important when one defends one of the discussed positions, or any other ethical position for that matter, is that, first of all, one should decide for oneself whether one defends it as the correct ethical position or as a compromise. Second, one should take into account the costs of compromising, including the epistemic cost. This cost almost always provides a reason against compromising. Of course, this reason might be outweighed by reasons *for* compromising. However, even if this is so and one decides, after careful deliberation and taking into account the specific circumstances, to defend a compromise, one could still try to reduce the epistemic cost attached to compromise. One could do so by clearly stating that one defends the particular position as a compromise, at least if this does not defeat the purpose of doing so. Another way to reduce the cost is to try to keep arguments that are attempted at directly producing good policy or practice separate from one's arguments that aim support the correct position. For example, discussions in epistemic mode could be published in certain venues (for example, certain sections of academic journals), and discussions in advisory mode in others (for example, other sections of journals, or different journals). This would reduce the risk of weakening one's own and others' epistemic virtues, but it may also help to prevent compromise mistakenly being taken for an epistemically correct position. It would thus help to prevent the epistemic erosion of the debate.

But these are issues that need not detain me further here, for in writing this book, I have placed myself squarely in the epistemic mode. This book is not meant to offer policy advice. It is meant to help us get closer to the correct ethical position on the permissibility of embryonic stem cell research.

Bibliography

Abelson, Raziel, 'Moral Distance: What do we Owe to Unknown Strangers?', *Philosophical Forum*, 36 (2005), 31–9.

Annas, George J., 'A French Homunculus in a Tennessee Court', *Hastings Center Report*, 19 (1989), 20–2.

Annas, George J., Arthur Caplan, and Sherman Elias, 'Stem Cell Politics, Ethics and Medical Progress', *Nature Medicine*, 5 (1999), 1339–41.

Annis, David B., 'Abortion and the Potentiality Principle', *Southern Journal of Philosophy*, 22 (1984), 155–63.

Aquinas, Thomas, *Summa Theologica* II-II, q. 64, art. 7, 'Of Killing', in Richard J. Regan and William P. Baumgarth (eds), *On Law, Morality, and Politics* (Indianapolis, Ind., and Cambridge: Hackett Publishing Co, 1988).

Arkes, Hadley, et al., 'Production of Pluripotent Stem Cells by Oocyte-Assisted Reprogramming: Joint Statement with Signatories', *National Catholic Bioethics Quarterly*, 5 (2005), 579–83.

Assady, Suheir, et al., 'Insulin Production by Human Embryonic Stem Cells', *Diabetes*, 50 (2001), 1691–7.

Baker, Monya, 'iPS Cells: Potent Stuff', *Nature Methods*, 7 (2010), 17–19.

Barbagallo, Ignazio, et al., 'Overexpression of Heme Oxygenase-1 Increases Human Osteoblast Stem Cell Differentiation', *Journal of Bone and Mineral Metabolism*, 28 (2010), 276–88.

Beauchamp, Tom L., and James F. Childress, *Principles of Biomedical Ethics* (New York: Oxford University Press, 2001).

Beilhack, Georg F., et al., 'Purified Allogeneic Hematopoietic Stem Cell Transplantation Blocks Diabetes Pathogenesis in NOD Mice', *Diabetes*, 52 (2003), 59–68.

Belmonte, Juan Carlos Izpisúa, et al., 'Induced Pluripotent Stem Cells and Reprogramming: Seeing the Science through the Hype', *Nature Review Genetics*, 10 (2009), 878–83.

Braybrooke, David, 'The Possibilities of Compromise', *Ethics*, 93 (1982), 139–50.

Brevini, T. A. L., and F. Gandolfi, 'Parthenotes as a Source of Embryonic Stem Cells', *Cell Proliferation*, 41 (2008), 20–30.

Brock, Dan W., 'Truth or Consequences: The Role of Philosophers in Policy-Making', *Ethics*, 97 (1987), 786–91.

Brock, Dan W., 'Is a Consensus Possible on Stem Cell Research? Moral and Political Obstacles', *Journal of Medical Ethics*, 32 (2006), 36–42.

Brock, Dan W., 'Creating Embryos for Use in Stem Cell Research', *Journal of Law and Medical Ethics*, 38 (2010), 229-37.

Brown, Mark T., 'Moral Complicity in Induced Pluripotent Stem Cell Research', *Kennedy Institute of Ethics Journal*, 19 (2009), 1-22.

Bruce, Donald, 'Parthenogenetic Embryos don't Solve Embryo Ethical Problems', press release, Feb. 2002, <http://archive.srtp.org.uk/clonin79.htm>.

Burke, William J., et al., 'Stemming the Tide of Cloning', *First Things*, 158 (2005), 6-12.

Byrnes, W. Malcolm, 'The Flawed Scientific Basis of the Altered Nuclear Transfer-Oocyte Assisted Reprogramming (ANT-OAR) Proposal', *Stem Cell Review*, 1 (2007), 60-5.

Charo, Alta R., 'Every Cell is Sacred', in Paul Lauritzen (ed.), *Cloning and the Future of Human Embryo Research* (Oxford: Oxford University Press, 2001), 82-9.

Chin, Mark H., et al., 'Induced Pluripotent Stem Cells and Embryonic Stem Cells are Distinguished by Gene Expression Signatures', *Cell Stem Cell*, 5 (2009), 111-23.

Christian Telegraph, 'Science: Adult Stem Cells More Promising than Embryonic', accessed Feb. 2014, <http://www.christiantelegraph.com/issue7717.html>.

Cibelli, Jose B., Kerrianne Cunniff, and Kent E. Vrana, 'Embryonic Stem Cells from Parthenotes', *Methods in Enzymology*, 418 (2006), 117-35.

Cibelli, Jose B., 'Is Therapeutic Cloning Dead?', *Science*, 318 (2007), 1879-80.

Cohen, G. A., 'Incentives, Inequality and Community', The Tanner Lectures on Human Values, delivered at Stanford University, May 1991.

Colombo, Roberto, 'Altered Nuclear Transfer', *Communio*, 31 (2004), 645-8.

Commission of the European Communities, *Commission Staff Working Paper: Report on Human Embryonic Stem Cell Research* (Brussels: Commission of the European Communities, 2003).

Committee of Inquiry into Human Fertilisation and Embryology, *The 'Warnock Report'* (London: Her Majesty's Stationery Office, 1978).

Condic, Maureen L., Patrick Lee, and Robert P. George, 'Ontological and Ethical Implications of Direct Nuclear Reprogramming: Response to Magill and Neaves', *Kennedy Institute of Ethics Journal*, 19 (2009), 33-40.

Congress, t. 1995 H. R. 2127; 1404 H. R. 2127. C. o. A. House of Representatives (1995).

Cowan, Chad A., Jocelyn Atienza, Douglas A. Melton, and Kevin Eggan, 'Nuclear Reprogramming of Somatic Cells After Fusion with Human Embryonic Stem Cells', *Science*, 309 (2005), 1369-73.

Daley, George Q., et al., 'Broader Implications of Defining Standards for the Pluripotency of iPSCs', *Cell Stem Cell*, 4 (2009), 200-20.

Darwall, Stephen L., 'Two Kinds of Respect', *Ethics*, 88 (1977), 36–49.

Davis, Dena S., 'Embryos Created for Research Purposes', *Kennedy Institute of Ethics Journal*, 5 (1995), 343–54.

Denker, Hans-Werner, 'Potentiality of Embryonic Stem Cells: An Ethical Problem Even with Alternative Stem Cell Sources', *Journal of Medical Ethics*, 32 (2006), 665–71.

Denker, Hans-Werner, 'Induced Pluripotent Stem Cells: How to Deal with the Developmental Potential', *Reproductive BioMedicine Online*, 19 (2009), 34–7.

Department of Health and Human Services and National Institutes of Health, *Plan for Implementation of Executive Order 13435: Expanding Approved Stem Cell Lines in Ethically Responsible Ways*, 18 Sept. 2007, <http://stemcells.nih. gov/staticresources/policy/eo13435.pdf>.

Deutsche Forschungsgemeinschaft (German Research Foundation), 'New DFG Recommendations Concerning Research with Human Stem Cells', press release 16 (3 May 2001).

Devolder, Katrien, and John Harris, 'The Ambiguity of the Embryo: Ethical Inconsistency in the Human Embryonic Stem Cell Debate', *Metaphilosophy*, 28/2–3 (2007), 153–69.

Devolder, Katrien, and Christopher M. Ward, 'Rescuing Human Embryonic Stem Cell Research: The Possibility of Embryo Reconstitution', *Metaphilosophy*, 28 (2007), 245–63.

Devolder, Katrien, 'Embryo Deaths in Reproduction and Embryo Research: A Reply to Murphy's Double Effect Argument', *Journal of Medical Ethics* (2012), doi:10.1136/medethics-2012-101065.

Devolder, Katrien, 'Killing Discarded Embryos and the Nothing-is-Lost Principle', *Journal of Applied Philosophy*, 30 (2013), 289–303.

Devolder, Katrien, 'To Be, or Not to Be?', *EMBO Reports*, 10 (2009), 1285–7.

de Wert, Guido, and Christine Mummery, 'Human Embryonic Stem Cells: Research, Ethics and Policy', *Human Reproduction*, 18 (2003), 672–82.

Doerflinger, Richard M., 'The Ethics of Funding Embryonic Stem Cell Research: A Catholic Viewpoint', *Kennedy Institute of Ethics Journal*, 9 (1999), 137–50.

Donagan, Alan, *The Theory of Morality* (Chicago: University of Chicago Press, 1977).

ESHRE Taskforce on Ethics and Law, 'Stem Cells', *Human Reproduction*, 17 (2002), 1409–10.

Feki, Anis, et al., 'Derivation of the First Swiss Human Embryonic Stem Cell Line from a Single Blastomere of an Arrested Four-Cell-Stage Embryo', *Swiss Medical Weekly*, 138 (2009), 640–60.

FitzPatrick, William, 'Surplus Embryos, Nonreproductive Cloning, and the Intend/Foresee Distinction', *Hastings Center Report*, 33 (2003), 29–36.

Fleck, Leonard M., 'Abortion, Deformed Fetuses, and the Omega Pill', *Philosophical Studies*, 36 (1979), 271–83.

Fletcher, Joseph C., 'NBAC's Arguments on Embryo Research: Strengths and Weaknesses', in Suzanne Holland, Karen Lebacqz, and Laurie Zoloth (eds), *The Human Embryonic Stem Cell Debate: Science, Ethics, and Public Policy* (Cambridge, Mass.: MIT Press, 2001), 61–72.

Frist, Bill, *A Senator Speaks Out on Ethics, Respect, and Compassion* (Washington, DC: Monument Press, 2005).

Gavrilov, Svetlana, Virginia E. Papaioannou, and Donald W. Landry, 'Alternative Strategies for the Derivation of Human Embryonic Stem Cell Lines and the Role of Dead Embryos', *Current Stem Cell Research and Therapy*, 4 (2009), 81–6.

Gerami-Naini, Behzad, et al., 'Trophoblast Differentiation in Embryoid Bodies Derived from Human Embryonic Stem Cells', *Endocrinology*, 145 (2004), 1517–24.

Gillam, Lynn, 'Arguing by Analogy in the Fetal Tissue Debate', *Bioethics*, 11 (1997), 397–412.

Glover, Jonathan, and M. J. Scott-Taggart, 'It Makes No Difference Whether or Not I Do it', *Proceedings of the Aristotelian Society*, 49 (1975), 171–209.

Gómez-Lobo, Alfonso, 'Does Respect for Embryos Entail Respect for Gametes?', *Theoretical Medicine and Bioethics*, 25 (2004), 199–208.

Green, Ronald M., 'Benefiting from "Evil": An Incipient Moral Problem in Human Stem Cell Research', *Bioethics*, 16 (2002), 544–56.

Guenin, Louis M., 'A Failed Noncomplicity Scheme', *Stem Cells and Development*, 13 (2004), 456–9.

Guenin, Louis M., *The Morality of Embryo Use* (Cambridge: Cambridge University Press, 2008).

Hanna, Jacob et al., 'Treatment of Sickle Cell Anemia Mouse Model with iPS Cells Generated from Autologous Skin', *Science*, 318 (2007), 1920–3.

Harman, Elizabeth, 'How is the Ethics of Stem Cell Research Different from the Ethics of Abortion?', *Metaphilosophy*, 38 (2007), 207–25.

Harris, John, 'Sexual Reproduction is a Survival Lottery', *Cambridge Quarterly of Healthcare Ethics*, 13 (2004), 75–89.

Harun, R., et al., 'Cytotrophoblast Stem Cell Lines Derived from Human Embryonic Stem Cells and their Capacity to Mimic Invasive Implantation Events', *Human Reproduction*, 21 (2006), 1349–58.

Heinemann, Thomas, and Ludger Honnefelder, 'Principles of Ethical Decision Making Regarding Embryonic Stem Cell Research in Germany', *Bioethics*, 16 (2002), 530–43.

Holden, Constance, and Gretchen Vogel, 'A Seismic Shift for Stem Cell Research', *Science* 319 (2008), 560–3.

Holland, Stephen, *Bioethics: A Philosophical Introduction* (Oxford: Polity, 2002).

Holm, Søren, 'The Ethical Case against Stem Cell Research', *Cambridge Quarterly of Healthcare Ethics*, 12 (2003), 372–83.

Holm, Søren, '"New Embryos": New Challenges for the Ethics of Stem Cell Research', *Cells Tissues Organs*, 187 (2008), 257–62.

House of Lords, Select Committee on Stem Cell Research, *Stem Cell Research: Report* (London: The House of Lords, 2002).

Hu, Bao-Yang, et al., 'Neural Differentiation of Human Induced Pluripotent Stem Cells Follows Developmental Principles But with Variable Potency', *Proceedings of the National Academy of Sciences USA*, 107 (2010), 4335–40.

Hug, Kristina, and Göran Hermerén, 'Do we Still Need Human Embryonic Stem Cells for Stem Cell-Based Therapies? Epistemic and Ethical Aspects', *Stem Cell Reviews and Reports*, 7 (2011), 761–74.

Hurlbut, William B., 'Altered Nuclear Transfer as a Morally Acceptable Means for the Procurement of Human Embryonic Stem Cells', 3 Dec. 2004, <http://bioethics.georgetown.edu/pcbe/background/hurlbut.html>.

Hurlbut, William B., 'Altered Nuclear Transfer as a Morally Acceptable Means for the Procurement of Human Embryonic Stem Cells', *Perspectives in Biology and Medicine*, 48 (2005), 211–28.

Ilic, Dusko, et al., 'Effect of Karyotype on Successful Human Embryonic Stem Cell Derivation', *Stem Cells and Development*, 19 (2010), 39–46.

Jensen, Gitte S., and Christian Drapeau, 'The Use of in situ Bone Marrow Stem Cells for the Treatment of Various Degenerative Diseases', *Medical Hypotheses*, 59 (2002), 422–8.

Jong-Hoon, Kim, et al., 'Dopamine Neurons Derived from Embryonic Stem Cells Function in an Animal Model of Parkinson's Disease', *Nature*, 418 (2002), 50–6.

Kagan, Shelly, 'Do I Make a Difference?', *Philosophy and Public Affairs* 39 (2011), 105–41.

Kahn, Axel, 'Clone Mammals . . . Clone Man?', *Nature*, 336 (1997), 119.

Kahn, Axel, 'Cloning, Dignity and Ethical Revisionism', *Nature*, 388 (1997), 320.

Kang, Lan, et al., 'iPS Cells Can Support Full-Term Development of Tetraploid Blastocyst-Complemented Embryos', *Cell Stem Cell*, 5 (2009), 135–8.

Kehat, Izhak, et al., 'Human Embryonic Stem Cells Can Differentiate into Myocytes with Structural and Functional Properties of Cardiomyocytes', *Journal of Clinical Investigation*, 108 (2001), 407–14.

Klimanskaya, Irina, et al., 'Human Embryonic Stem Cell Lines Derived from Single Blastomeres', *Nature*, 444 (2006), 481–5.

Krauthammer, Charles, 'Stem Cell Vindication for Bush', *Washington Post*, 30 Nov. 2007, A23, <http://www.washingtonpost.com/wp-dyn/content/article/2007/11/29/AR2007112901878.html>.

Kuhse, Helga, and Peter Singer, 'The Moral Status of the Embryo', in William A. W. Walters and Peter Singer (eds). *Test-Tube Babies: A Guide to Moral Questions, Present Techniques, and Future Possibilities* (Melbourne: Oxford University Press, 1982), 57–63.

Kuhse, Helga, and Peter Singer, 'Individuals, Humans, and Persons: The Issue of Moral Status' in Peter Singer and Helga Kuhse (eds), *Unsanctifying Human Life: Essays on Ethics* (Oxford: Wiley-Blackwell, 2002), 188–98.

Landry, Donald W., and Howard A. Zucker, 'Embryonic Death and the Creation of Human Embryonic Stem Cells', *Journal of Clinical Investigation*, 114 (2004), 1184–6.

Lerou, Paul H., et al., 'Human Embryonic Stem Cell Derivation from Poor-Quality Embryos', *Nature Biotechnology*, 26 (2008), 212–14.

Levenberg, Shulamit, et al., 'Endothelial Cells Derived from Human Embryonic Stem Cells', *Proceedings of the National Academy of Sciences USA*, 99 (2002), 4391–6.

Li, Wenlin, et al., 'Generation of Rat and Human Induced Pluripotent Stem Cells by Combining Genetic Reprogramming and Chemical Inhibitors', *Cell Stem Cell*, 4 (2009), 16–19.

Liao, Matthew S., 'Rescuing Human Embryonic Stem Cell Research: The Blastocyst Transfer Method', *American Journal of Bioethics*, 5 (2005), 8–16.

Liao, Matthew S., 'The Embryo Rescue Case', *Theoretical Medicine and Bioethics*, 27 (2006), 141–7.

Lin, Ge, et al., 'A Highly Homozygous and Parthenogenetic Human Embryonic Stem Cell Line Derived from a One-Pronuclear Oocyte Following in vitro Fertilization Procedure', *Cell Research*, 17 (2007), 999–1007.

Lu, Bin, et al., 'Long-Term Safety and Function of RPE from Human Embryonic Stem Cells in Preclinical Models of Macular Degeneration', *Stem Cells*, 27 (2009), 2126–35.

Lui, Kathy O., Herman Waldmann, and Paul J. Fairchild, 'Embryonic Stem Cells: Overcoming the Immunological Barriers to Cell Replacement Therapy', *Current Stem Cell Research and Therapy*, 4 (2009), 70–80.

Lund, Raymond D., et al., 'Human Embryonic Stem Cell–Derived Cells Rescue Visual Function in Dystrophic RCS Rats', *Cloning and Stem Cells*, 8 (2006), 189–99.

Lysaught, M. Therese, 'Respect: Or, How Respect for Persons Became Respect for Autonomy', *Journal of Medicine and Philosophy*, 29 (2004), 665–80.

Macchiarini, Paolo, et al., 'Clinical Transplantation of a Tissue-Engineered Airway', *The Lancet*, 372 (2008), 2023–30.

McCormick, Jennifer B., Jason Owen-Smith, and Christopher Thomas Scott, 'Distribution of Human Embryonic Stem Cell Lines: Who, When, and Where', *Cell Stem Cell*, 4 (2009), 107–10.

Magill, Gerard, and William B. Neaves, 'Ontological and Ethical Implications of Direct Nuclear Reprogramming', *Kennedy Institute of Ethics Journal*, 19 (2009), 23–32.

Mai, Qingyun, et al., 'Derivation of Human Embryonic Stem Cell Lines from Parthenogenetic Blastocysts', *Cell Research*, 17 (2007), 1008–19.

Mangan, Joseph, 'An Historical Analysis of the Principle of Double Effect', *Theological Studies*, 10 (1949), 41–61.

Marquis, Don, 'Why Abortion is Immoral', *Journal of Philosophy*, 86 (1989), 183–202.

McDonald, John W., et al., 'Transplanted Embryonic Stem Cells Survive, Differentiate and Promote Recovery in Injured Rat Spinal Cord', *Nature Medicine*, 5 (1999), 1410–12.

McHugh, Paul R., 'Zygote and "Clonote": The Ethical Use of Embryonic Stem Cells', *New England Journal of Medicine*, 351 (2004), 209–10.

McMahan, Jeff, *The Ethics of Killing: Problems at the Margins of Life* (New York: Oxford University Press, 2002).

Meissner, Alexander, and Rudolph Jaenisch, 'Generation of Nuclear Transfer-Derived Pluripotent ES Cells from Cloned Cdx2-Deficient Blastocysts', *Nature*, 439 (2006), 212–15.

Melton, Douglas A., George Q. Daley, and Charles G. Jennings, 'Altered Nuclear Transfer in Stem-Cell Research: A Flawed Proposal', *New England Journal of Medicine* 351 (2004), 2791–2.

Mertes, Heidi, and Guido Pennings, 'Stem Cell Research Policies: Who's Afraid of Complicity?', *Reproductive BioMedicine Online*, 19 (2009), 38–42.

Meyer, John R., 'Human Embryonic Stem Cells and Respect for Life', *Journal of Medical Ethics*, 26 (2000), 166–70.

Meyer, John R., 'The Significance of Induced Pluripotent Stem Cells for Basic Research and Clinical Therapy', *Journal of Medical Ethics*, 3 (2008), 849–51.

Meyer, Michael J., and Lawrence J. Nelson, 'Respecting What we Destroy: Reflections on Human Embryo Research', *Hastings Center Report*, 31 (2001), 16–23.

Min, Jiang-Yong, et al., 'Transplantation of Embryonic Stem Cells Improves Cardiac Function in Postinfarcted Rats', *Journal of Applied Physiology*, 92 (2002), 288–96.

Moraczewski, Albert S., 'May one Benefit from the Evil Deeds of Others?', *National Catholic Bioethics Quarterly*, 2 (2002), 43–7.

Moschidou, Dafni, et al., 'Valproic Acid Confers Functional Pluripotency to Human Amniotic Fluid Stem Cells in a Transgene-Free Approach', *Molecular Therapy*, 20 (2012), 1953–67.

Murphy, Timothy M., 'Double-Effect Reasoning and the Conception of Human Embryos', *Journal of Medical Ethics*, 2012, doi:10.1136/medethics-2012-100534.

Nagy, Andras, et al., 'Embryonic Stem Cells Alone are Able to Support Foetal Development in the Mouse', *Development*, 110 (1990), 815–21.

National Advisory Bioethics Commission, *Ethical Issues in Human Stem Cell Research* (Rockville, MD: NBAC, 1999).

National Institutes of Health, Ad Hoc Group of Consultants to the Advisory Committee to the Director, *Report of the Human Embryo Research Panel* (Washington, DC: NIH, 1994).

Ord, Toby, 'The Scourge: Moral Implications of Natural Embryo Loss', *American Journal of Bioethics*, 8 (2008), 12–19.

Outka, Gene, 'The Ethics of Human Stem Cell Research', *Kennedy Institute of Ethics Journal*, 12 (2002), 175–213.

Outka, Gene, 'The Ethics of Embryonic Stem Cell Research and the Principle of Nothing is Lost', *Yale Journal of Health Policy Law and Ethics*, 9 (2009), 585–602.

Parfit, Derek, *Reasons and Persons* (Oxford: Oxford University Press, 1984).

Park, Jennifer S., et al., 'The Effect of Matrix Stiffness on the Differentiation of Mesenchymal Stem Cells in Response to TGF- b', *Biomaterials*, 32 (2011), 3921–30.

Pellestor, F., B. Andreo, T. Anahory, and S. Hamamah, 'The Occurrence of Aneuploidy in Human: Lessons from the Cytogenetic Studies of Human Oocytes', *European Journal of Medical Genetics*, 49 (2006), 103–16.

Pennings, Guido, and André Van Steirteghem, 'The Subsidiarity Principle in the Context of Embryonic Stem Cell Research', *Human Reproduction*, 19 (2004), 1060–4.

Pilar, Cervera Rita, and Miodrag Stojkovic, 'Commentary: Somatic Cell Nuclear Transfer: Progress and Promise', *Stem Cells*, 26 (2008), 494–5.

Plath, Kathrin, and William E. Lowry, 'Progress in Understanding Reprogramming to the Induced Pluripotent State', *Nature Review Genetics*, 12 (2011), 253–65.

President's Council on Bioethics, *Human Cloning and Human Dignity: An Ethical Inquiry* (Washington, DC: President's Council on Bioethics, 2002).

President's Council on Bioethics, *Alternative Sources of Pluripotent Stem Cells* (Washington, DC: President's Council on Bioethics, May 2005).

Prieur, Michael R., et al., 'Stem Cell Research in a Catholic Institution: Yes or No?', *Kennedy Institute of Ethics Journal*, 16 (2006), 73–98.

Pugh, Jonathan, 'Is the "Compromise Position" Concerning the Moral Permissibility of Different Forms of Human Embryonic Stem Cell Research a Tenable Position?' (MSc thesis, University of Edinburgh, 2010).

Pugh, Jonathan, 'Embryos, The Principle of Proportionality, and the Shaky Ground of Moral Respect', *Bioethics* 2013 doi: 10.1111/bioe.12013.

Rabb, Harriet S., Letter to H. Varmus (NIH), 'Federal Funding for Research Involving Human Pluripotent Stem Cells', General Council, Washington, DC, 15 Jan. 1999.

Rao, Mahendra, and Maureen L. Condic, 'Alternative Sources of Pluripotent Stem Cells', *Stem Cells and Development*, 17 (2008), 1–10.

Reubinoff, Benjamin E., et al., 'Embryonic Stem Cell Lines from Human Blastocysts: Somatic Differentiation in Vitro', *Nature Biotechnology*, 18 (2000), 399–404.

Revazova, Elena S., et al., 'HLA Homozygous Stem Cell Lines Derived from Human Parthenogenetic Blastocysts: Cloning Stem Cells', *Cloning Stem Cells*, 9 (2007), 432–49.

Rideout, William M., et al., 'Correction of a Genetic Defect by Nuclear Transplantation and Combined Cell and Gene Therapy', *Cell*, 109 (2002), 17–27.

Robertson, John A., 'Causative vs. Beneficial Complicity in the Embryonic Stem Cell Debate', *Connecticut Law Review*, 36 (2003), 1099–113.

Robinton, Daisy A., and George Q. Daley, 'The Promise of Induced Pluripotent Stem Cells in Research and Therapy', *Nature*, 481 (2012), 295–305.

Sampaolesi, Maurilio, et al. 'Mesoangioblast Stem Cells Ameliorate Muscle Function in Dystrophic Dogs', *Nature*, 444 (2006), 574–9.

Savulescu, Julian, 'Should we Clone Human Beings? Cloning as a Source of Tissue for Transplantation', *Journal of Medical Ethics* 25 (1999), 87–95.

Savulescu, Julian, 'The Embryonic Stem Cell Lottery and the Cannibalization of Human Beings', *Bioethics*, 16 (2002), 508–29.

Schindler, David L., 'A Response to the Joint Statement, "Production of Pluripotent Stem Cells by Oocyte Assisted Reprogramming"', *Communio*, 32 (Summer 2005), 369–80.

Scott, Christopher Thomas, et al., 'Democracy Derived? New Trajectories in Pluripotent Stem Cell Research', *Cell*, 145 (2011), 820–6.

Shah, Ramille N., et al., 'Supramolecular Design of Self-Assembling Nanofibers for Cartilage Regeneration', *Proceedings of the National Academy of Sciences*, 107 (2010), 3293–8.

Singer, Peter, 'Famine, Affluence, and Morality', *Philosophy and Public Affairs*, 1 (1972), 229–43.

Singer, Peter, 'A Vegetarian Philosophy', in Sian Griffiths and Jennifer Wallace (eds), *Consuming Passions* (Manchester: Manchester University Press, 1998), 66–72.

Singer, Peter, and Karen Dawson, 'IVF Technology and the Argument from Potential', *Philosophy and Public Affairs*, 17 (1988), 87–104.

Solter, Davor, Deryck Beyleveld, and Minou Friele. *Embryo Research in Pluralistic Europe* (Berlin and Heidelberg: Springer-Verlag, 2003).

Soria, Bernat, et al., 'Insulin-Secreting Cells Derived from Embryonic Stem Cells Normalize Glycemia in Streptozotocin-Induced Diabetic Mice', *Diabetes*, 49 (2000), 157–62.

Sparrow, Robert, and David Cram, 'Saviour Embryos? Preimplantation Genetic Diagnosis as a Therapeutic Technology', *Reproductive BioMedicine Online*, 20 (2010), 667–74.

Steinbock, Bonnie, 'What does "Respect for Embryos" Mean in the Context of Stem Cell Research?', *Women's Health Issues*, 10 (2000), 127–30.

Stier, Marco, and Bettina Schoene-Seifert, 'The Argument from Potentiality in the Embryo Protection Debate: Finally "Depotentialized"?', *American Journal of Bioethics*, 13 (2013), 19–27.

Strong, Carson, 'The Moral Status of Preembryos, Embryos, Foetuses, and Infants', *Journal of Medicine and Philosophy*, 22 (1997), 457–78.

Strong, Carson, 'Obtaining Stem Cells: Moving from Scylla toward Charybdis', *American Journal of Bioethics*, 5 (2005), 21–3.

Suaudeau, J., 'From Embryonic Stem Cells to iPS: An Ethical Perspective', *Cell Proliferation*, 44 (2011), 70–84.

Sumner, L. W., *Abortion and Moral Theory* (Princeton: Princeton University Press, 1981).

Takahashi, Kazutoshi, and Shinya Yamanaka, 'Induction of Pluripotent Stem Cells from Mouse Embryonic and Adult Fibroblast Cultures by Defined Factors', *Cell*, 126 (2006), 663–76.

Takahashi, Kazutoshi, et al., 'Induction of Pluripotent Stem Cells from Adult Human Fibroblasts by Defined Factors', *Cell*, 131 (2007), 861–72.

Takala, Tuija, and Matti Häyry, 'Benefiting from Past Wrongdoing, Human Embryonic Stem Cell Lines, and the Fragility of the German Legal Position', *Bioethics*, 21 (2007), 150–9.

Taylor, Craig J., et al., 'Banking on Human Embryonic Stem Cells: Estimating the Number of Donor Cell Lines Needed for HLA Matching', *The Lancet*, 366 (2005), 2019–25.

Testa, Guiseppe, 'Stem Cells through Stem Beliefs: The Co-Production of Bio-technological Pluralism', *Science as Culture*, 17 (2008), 435–48.

Testa, Giuseppe, Lodovica Borghese, Julius A. Steinbeck, and Oliver Brüstle, 'Breakdown of the Potentiality Principle and its Impact on Global Stem Cell Research', *Cell Stem Cell*, 1 (2007), 153–6.

Thomson, James A., et al., 'Embryonic Stem Cell Lines Derived from Human Blastocysts', *Science*, 282 (1998), 1145–7.

Thomson, Judith Jarvis, 'A Defense of Abortion', *Philosophy and Public Affairs*, 1 (1977), 47–66.

Urbach, Achia, et al., 'Differential Modeling of Fragile X Syndrome by Human Embryonic Stem Cells and Induced Pluripotent Stem Cells', *Cell Stem Cell*, 6 (2010), 407–11.

US Conference of Catholic Bishops, *On Embryonic Stem Cell Research: A Statement of the United States Conference of Catholic Bishops*, 2008,

<http://stemcell.www65.a2hosting.com/wp-content/uploads/2013/11/usccb_2008-06-13.pdf>.

US Government, *Executive Order 13435: Expanding Approved Stem Cell Lines in Ethically Responsible Ways* (Federal Register, 22 June 2007), 34951–3, <http://edocket.access.gpo.gov/2007/pdf/07-3112.pdf>.

Verlinsky Yuri, et al., 'Preimplantation Diagnosis for Immunodeficiencies', *Reproductive BioMedicine Online*, 14 (2007), 214–23.

Watt, Helen, 'Potential and the Early Human', *Journal of Medical Ethics*, 22 (1996), 222–6.

White House. Office of the Press Secretary. 'Radio address by the President to the nation', Bush Ranch, Tex., 11 Aug. 2001, <http://www.whitehouse.gov/news/releases/2001/08/20010809-2.html>.

White House, Office of the Press Secretary, *Executive Order: Removing Barriers to Responsible Scientific Research Involving Human Stem Cells*, 9 Mar. 2009, <http://www.whitehouse.gov/the-press-office/removing-barriers-responsible-scientific-research-involving-human-stem-cells>.

Williams, Bernard A. O., 'A Critique of Utilitarianism', in J. J. C. Smart and Bernard A. O. Williams (eds) *Utilitarianism: For and Against* (Cambridge: Cambridge University Press, 1973), 82–117.

Yu, Junying, et al., 'Induced Pluripotent Stem Cell Lines Derived from Human Somatic Cells', *Science*, 318 (2007), 1917–20.

Zhang, Xin, et al., 'Derivation of Human Embryonic Stem Cells from Developing and Arrested Embryos', *Stem Cells*, 24 (2006), 2669–76.

Zhao, Xiao-yang, et al., 'iPS Cells Produce Viable Mice through Tetraploid Complementation', *Nature*, 461 (2009), 86–90.

Index